FAST FACTS

FF

Indispensable
Guides to
Clinical
Practice

Respiratory Tract Infection

Second edition

Robert C Read
Honorary Consultant Physician
and Professor of Infectious Diseases,
Royal Hallamshire Hospital,
Sheffield, UK

Donald E Craven
Professor of Medicine,
Tufts University School of Medicine,
Boston, Massachusetts;
Chair, Department of Infectious Diseases,
Lahey Clinic, Burlington,
Massachusetts, USA

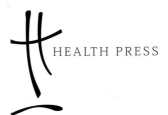

HEALTH PRESS

Oxford

Fast Facts – Respiratory Tract Infection
First published 1998
Second edition January 2003

Text © 2003 Robert C Read, Donald E Craven
© 2003 in this edition Health Press Limited
Health Press Limited, Elizabeth House, Queen Street,
Abingdon, Oxford OX14 3JR, UK
Tel: +44 (0)1235 523233
Fax: +44 (0)1235 523238

Fast Facts is a trademark of Health Press Limited

The publisher and the authors have made every effort to ensure the
accuracy of this book, but cannot accept responsibility for any errors or
omissions.

A CIP catalogue record for this title is available from the British Library.

ISBN 1-903734-22-3

Read, RC (Robert C)
Fast Facts – Respiratory Tract Infection/
Robert C Read, Donald E Craven

Medical illustrations by Jane Fallows, London, UK.

Typesetting and page layout by Zed, Oxford, UK.

Printed by Fine Print (Services) Ltd, Oxford, UK.

PHS

Glossary of abbreviations

ABPA: allergic bronchopulmonary aspergillosis

AFB: acid-fast bacilli

APACHE: acute physiology and chronic health evaluation

ARDS: adult respiratory distress syndrome

BAL: bronchoalveolar lavage

CAP: community-acquired pneumonia

CFTR: cystic fibrosis transmembrane regulator (protein)

CMV: cytomegalovirus

COPD: chronic obstructive pulmonary disease

CPIS: clinical pulmonary infection score

CSF: cerebrospinal fluid

CT: computed tomography

DIC:, diffuse intravascular coagulation

DLCO: diffusing capacity for carbon monoxide

DOTS: directly observed therapy, short course

FEV$_1$: forced expiratory volume in 1 second

FNA: fine-needle aspirate

FVC: forced vital capacity

GNB: Gram-negative bacteria

HAP: hospital-acquired pneumonia

HAART: highly active antiretroviral therapy

HIV: human immunodeficiency virus

HRCT: high-resolution computed tomography

HSV: herpes simplex virus

ICU: intensive care unit

IFA: immunofluorescence assay

IFN: interferon

KS: Kaposi's sarcoma

MDR: multi-drug-resistant

MIC: minimum inhibitory concentration

MRSA: methicillin-resistant *S. aureus*

NPA: nasopharyngeal aspirate

PCP: *Pneumocystis carinii* pneumonia

PCR: polymerase chain reaction

PEF: peak expiratory flow

PSB: protected specimen brush

PSI: pulmonary severity of illness

QEA: quantitative endotracheal aspirates

SIRS: systemic inflammatory response syndrome

TB: tuberculosis

TNF: tumor necrosis factor

VAP: ventilator-associated pneumonia

VRE: vancomycin-resistant enterococci

1 Community-acquired pneumonia

Pneumonia is a general term used to describe disease that leads to consolidation of the lung parenchyma. It is characterized by acute inflammation within the gas-exchanging areas of the lung with an intense infiltrate of neutrophils in and around the alveoli and the respiratory and terminal bronchioles. The affected bronchopulmonary segment or the entire lobe may be consolidated by the resulting inflammation and edema.

Epidemiology

In the UK, the rate of hospital admissions for pneumonia is approximately 1/1000/year. In the USA, the prevalence is estimated to be 12/1000/year (i.e. approximately 3.3 million cases/year), and bacterial pneumonias account for 500 000 hospital admissions/year of patients aged 15 years or older.

Pneumonia is substantially more common in the winter and affects males more often than females (ratio 2–3:1). It most commonly affects the elderly: in the USA, the incidence of pneumonia requiring hospitalization in those over 75 years of age is 11.6/1000/year, compared with 0.54/1000/year in those aged 35–44 years. Rates of pneumonia in the elderly are expected to double in the next 25 years.

Mortality and morbidity

Mortality due to community-acquired pneumonia (CAP) has decreased markedly since the introduction of antibiotics; the outcome for patients admitted to hospital with pneumonia can be greatly improved by prompt antibiotic therapy. Mortality from ambulatory pneumonia is now about 1% (ambulatory pneumonia is that affecting outpatients/people in the community). In hospitalized patients, however, mortality is approximately 13–15% and, in patients requiring intensive care, it ranges from 22% to 54%.

Patients who survive pneumonia generally recover completely, though there are occasionally long-term sequelae. Patients with sepsis syndrome, usually in association with *Streptococcus pneumoniae*, *Legionella pneumophila* or *Klebsiella pneumoniae* infections, often suffer significant morbidity.

Pathogenesis

Most infections result from initial colonization of the upper respiratory tract by a pathogen, with subsequent translocation by aspiration into the lower airways. The most common cause of community-acquired pneumonia is *S. pneumoniae*, but a wide range of other pathogens may also be implicated (Table 1.1).

Assessment and treatment

Clinical features. In most patients, pneumonia usually develops over several days with cough and sputum production, dyspnea, pleuritic chest pain, weakness, malaise and often myalgia. Occasionally, the presentation may be hyperacute with a dramatic rigor as the first symptom; this is more common in healthy young adults. In older patients, the presentation may be more insidious, with minimal cough and absence of fever; confusion and hypothermia are often presenting features in this group.

Physical examination usually reveals fever, particularly in young individuals. Patients are usually uncomfortable and may often be breathless at rest. The trachea is usually central, but expansion on the affected side is reduced. Percussion is dull over the diseased lobe or lobes, and auscultation may reveal rales or bronchial breathing, depending on the degree of consolidation. Occasionally, there is evidence of an effusion with stony dullness on the affected side. Typical chest radiographs are reproduced in Figures 1.1 and 1.2.

In pneumococcal pneumonia, the sputum is classically rust colored, but can be mucoid, scanty or absent. In *Mycoplasma*, *Chlamydia*, *Legionella* and viral infections, sputum is usually absent. Characteristic epidemiological and clinical features and laboratory abnormalities that may point to a specific microbiological diagnosis are listed in Table 1.2.

Investigations. Chest radiography is critical for establishing the diagnosis and for distinguishing pneumonia from acute bronchitis.

TABLE 1.1

Causes of community-acquired pneumonia

Pathogen	Cases (%)
Bacteria	
• *Streptococcus pneumoniae*	30–54
• *Haemophilus influenzae*	6–15
• *Staphylococcus aureus*	0–2
• *Klebsiella pneumoniae*	0–2
• Other *Streptococcus* spp.	0–1
• Enterobacteriaceae; *E. coli*, etc	0–1
• Anaerobes	variable
'Atypical' pathogens	
• *Mycoplasma pneumoniae*	0–18
• *Legionella pneumophila*	2–7
• *Chlamydia pneumoniae*	0–6
• *Chlamydia psittaci*	0–3
• *Coxiella burnetii*	0–1
Viruses	
• Influenza A virus	6–9
• Respiratory syncytial virus	0–1
• Hantavirus	0–1

Rare pathogens

Bacillus anthracis, Francisella tularensis, Yersinia pestis, Pneumocystis carinii, Histoplasma spp, *Cryptococcus* spp., *Mycobacterium tuberculosis, Nocardia* spp, *Neisseria meningitidis.*

Adapted in part from Meyer RD, Finch RG. *J Hosp Infect* 1992;22(Suppl A):51–9

Additional studies should be ordered if the patient requires hospitalization, as discussed below. Initial investigations for suspected pneumonia include:

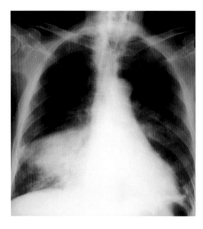

Figure 1.1 Right lower lobe consolidation in a 25-year-old male. *Streptococcus pneumoniae* was isolated in blood cultures.

Figure 1.2 Right upper lobe consolidation in a 42-year-old male with *Klebsiella pneumoniae* pneumonia. Note the bulging horizontal fissure.

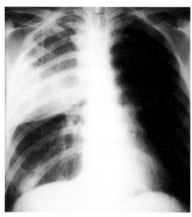

- routine hematology and biochemistry
- blood cultures
- chest radiograph
- sputum examination and culture (if sputum is expectorated; Figure 1.3)
- cold agglutinins to detect *M. pneumoniae*
- pulse oximetry or blood gases
- acute and convalescent serology to detect antibodies to viruses (including hantaviruses in some localities), *Mycoplasma*, *Chlamydia*, *Legionella* and *Coxiella burnetii*
- urine antigen detection to detect *Legionella* antigen
- aspiration of pleural fluid (for biochemistry and culture).

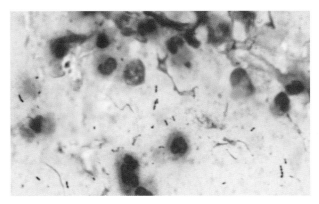

Figure 1.3 Gram stain of sputum from a patient with pneumococcal pneumonia showing pus cells and lanceolate Gram-positive cocci.

Risk stratification, site of treatment and mortality. When assessing a patient with pneumonia, it is important initially to assess the severity of the patient's disease and to determine whether the patient requires hospitalization or if outpatient management is possible. If hospitalization is necessary, the severity of disease will determine the initial selection of antibiotics to be given in the emergency room and the need for care in the intensive care unit (ICU).

Recently, a prediction rule using a scoring system to help assess the patient's pulmonary severity of illness index (PSI) was published. Severity points are assigned by age, underlying disease, and severity of acute illness, based on clinical and laboratory parameters (Table 1.3). The PSI helps clinicians identify patients who can be safely managed as outpatients (Classes I–III) and those with severe disease who should be treated as inpatients on the medical ward or stabilized rapidly in the ICU (Classes IV–V). The total PSI point score correlates with patient mortality and stratifies patients by risk: low (Classes I–III), moderate (Class IV) or high risk (Class V) (Table 1.4). The hospital admission decision tree by risk class is outlined in Figure 1.4. Note that psychosocial factors should be evaluated that may alter the management plan.

Mortality rates increase dramatically in patients with severe pneumonia. The criteria for severe pneumonia are summarized in Table 1.5, but the sensitivity of the criteria is increased if a patient has

TABLE 1.2

Characteristic clinical features of pathogens causing community-acquired pneumonia

Pathogen	Epidemiological features
Bacteria	
• Streptococcus pneumoniae	Most common cause of CAP
• Haemophilus influenzae	Affects children and the elderly, especially those in nursing homes
• Staphylococcus aureus	Recent influenza infection
• Klebsiella pneumoniae	Affects alcoholics and the elderly in nursing homes
• Anaerobes	Aspiration
Atypical pathogens	
• Mycoplasma pneumoniae	Occurs in 4-yearly cycles
• Legionella pneumophila	History of exposure to contaminated aerosols (e.g. hotel air conditioning, respiratory devices)
• Chlamydia pneumoniae	Affects children in educational institutions and elderly in nursing homes
• Chlamydia psittaci	Contact with infected psittacine birds
• Coxiella burnetii	History of contact with farm animals
Viruses	
• Influenza A virus	Annual winter epidemic

Characteristic clinical features	Characteristic laboratory findings
Unilobar disease, rigors, toxemia	Gram-positive lanceolate cocci in sputum, neutrophil leukocytosis
Symptoms preceded by coryza with sudden onset of pleuritic pain	Gram-negative coccobacilli in sputum
I.v. drug abuse, aggressive and cavitating pneumonia with pleural effusions	Gram-positive cocci in sputum with neutrophil leukocytosis
Aggressive pneumonia, bulging fissure on chest radiograph	Gram-negative bacilli in sputum
Fever, cough, purulent sputum, leukocytosis, focal consolidation or abscess	Mixed Gram-positive and -negative rods and cocci. Culture only sterile body fluids
Insidious onset, headache, malaise, myalgia, pharyngitis, otalgia, cough due to peribronchitis, multilobar involvement	Cold agglutinins, convalescent antibody rise
Gradual onset, malaise, lethargy, fever, headache, myalgia, dry cough, confusion, hallucinations	Hyponatremia, abnormal liver function tests, positive urinary antigen, convalescent antibody rise
Prolonged mild upper and lower respiratory tract symptoms	Convalescent antibody rise
Predominant headache and pleuritic pain, dry cough	Convalescent antibody rise
Fever, malaise, headache, dry cough, pleuritic pain, prolonged fever	Phase 2 antibody rise
High fever, pharyngitis, bibasal pneumonia	Convalescent antibody rise, positive culture or PCR of NPA or throat swab

(CONTINUED)

TABLE 1.2 (CONTINUED)

Pathogen	Epidemiological features
• Respiratory syncytial virus	Annual winter epidemics; more common in young children
• Hantavirus	Southwestern USA; affects campers, those in contact with rodent feces
Rare pathogens	
• *Bacillus anthracis*	Bioterrorism, inhaled
• *Yersinia pestis*	Bioterrorism, inhaled, person-to-person transmission
• *Francisella tularensis*	Bioterrorism, small outbreaks related to rodents

IFA, immunofluorescence assay; NPA, nasopharyngeal aspirate; PCR, polymerase chain reaction

one of the two major criteria (mechanical ventilation or severe sepsis) and 2/3 of the minor criteria (systolic blood pressure < 90 mmHg, multilobar involvement or PaO_2/FiO_2 < 250 mmHg).

Initial antimicrobial therapy. Several evidence-based guidelines and clinical pathways for initial antibiotic therapy and clinical management of CAP have been recently published by the American Thoracic Society (ATS), the Infectious Diseases Society of America (IDSA), the European Respiratory Society (ERS) and the British Thoracic Society (BTC). Clearly, a working knowledge of these guidelines should improve the quality of care and improve outcomes in patients with CAP.

Because the specific pathogen responsible for pneumonia is usually not known, most patients receive early, empiric, broad-spectrum, therapy. Appropriate antibiotic therapy should preferably be administered in the Emergency Room and certainly within 8 hours of entering the hospital. Early, appropriate antibiotic therapy will reduce mortality, complications and length of stay.

Recently published guidelines for antibiotic treatment of outpatients are summarized in Table 1.6. Consideration should also be given to the

Characteristic clinical features	Characteristic laboratory findings
Fever, dry cough, patchy infiltrations	Culture, IFA and PCR of NPA or respiratory secretions
Aggressive pneumonia and sepsis syndrome with hemoptysis	Detection of antibodies
Fever, malaise, dry cough, respiratory distress, shock, widened mediastinum, leukocytosis	Gram-positive bacilli in blood and sputum culture
Fever, malaise, cough, bloody sputum, shock, leukocytosis, consolidation or patchy infiltrates	Sputum – Gram-negative bipolar coccobacilli, blood/sputum/CSF culture
Fever, prostration, cough, focal pneumonia with hilar nodes	Cultures of blood/sputum – Gram-negative bacilli

ability to take oral medications, adherence factors and the support systems of the patient. Some clinicians also believe that the initial dose of antibiotic therapy should be given intravenously for some patients assigned to outpatient care.

For patients hospitalized with mild to moderate pneumonia, a parenteral second- or third-generation cephalosporin (cefuroxime or ceftriaxone) plus a macrolide, such as azithromycin, or a third- or fourth-generation fluoroquinolone, such as moxifloxacin, levofloxacin or gatifloxacin) are recommended (Table 1.7). Available data indicate that the 30-day mortality was significantly reduced in patients with pneumonia treated with a quinolone alone or a cephalosporin plus macrolide in comparison to those who received a cephalosporin alone. Because first- and second-generation quinolones, such as ciprofloxacin and ofloxacin, have decreased activity against pneumococci, they are not recommended. Furthermore, certain risk groups and the presence of some risk factors, such as aspiration of anaerobes, may require additional antimicrobial coverage as described in Tables 1.6 and 1.7.

In patients with severe pneumonia, every effort should be made initially to cover all potential pathogens. Selection of antibiotics for

TABLE 1.3

The Pulmonary Severity Index (PSI) scoring system*

Patient characteristics	Points
Demographic factors	
• Male	Age (years)
• Female	Age (years) – 10
• Nursing home resident	10
Comorbidities	
• Neoplastic disease	30
• Liver disease	20
• Congestive heart failure	10
• Cerebrovascular disease	10
• Renal disease	10
Physical examination findings	
• Altered mental status	20
• Respiratory rate ≥ 30 breaths/min	20
• Systolic blood pressure < 90 mmHg	20
• Temperature < 35°C (95°F) or ≥ 40°C (104°F)	15
• Pulse rate ≥ 125 beats/min	10
Laboratory findings	
• pH < 7.35	30
• Blood urea nitrogen > 10.7 mmol/L	20
• Sodium < 130 mEq/L	20
• Glucose > 13.9 mmol/L	10
• Hematocrit < 30%	10
• PO_2 < 60 mmHg; O_2 sat < 90%	10
• Pleural effusion	10
Total	**(see Table 1.4)**

* The total score is used to classify severity of disease and suggest a potential site for management (Table 1.4)
Adapted from Fine et al. 1997

TABLE 1.4

Risk class, mortality rates and recommended site of care

Risk class		Total PSI points	Mortality (%)	Recommended site of care
I	Low	–	0.1	Outpatient
II	Low	≤ 70	0.6	Outpatient
III	Low	71–90	2.8	Outpatient or brief inpatient
IV	Moderate	91–30	8.2	Inpatient
V	High	> 130	29.2	Inpatient

Taken from Fine et al. 1997

patients with severe pneumonia will depend on the risk of
Pseudomonas aeruginosa, methicillin-resistant *Staphylococcus aureus*
(MRSA), drug-resistant pneumococci, and other multi-drug-resistant
(MDR) pathogens. In such patients, a third- or fourth-generation
antipseudomonal cephalosporin, such as cefotaxime or cefepime, with
or without vancomycin for MRSA, is recommended. If Gram-negative
pneumonia or an unusual pathogen such as *F. tularensis* is suspected in
a severely ill patient, the addition of an aminoglycoside, such as
gentamicin, tobramycin or amikacin is strongly suggested. Empiric
coverage for *Legionella*, *Mycoplasma* and *Chlamydia* with a quinolone
or macrolide (azithromycin or erythromycin) is also recommended
for patients with severe pneumonia. In patients with confirmed
L. pneumophila infection, use of intravenous erythromycin and
possibly the addition of rifampin (rifampicin in the UK) should be
considered. Anaerobe coverage is imperative in patients suspected
of aspiration or when there is suggestive evidence on the sputum
Gram stain. Once a definitive diagnosis is established and antibiotic
sensitivities are known, the broad-spectrum, empiric regimen can
often be narrowed.

Penicillin and multi-drug-resistant pneumococci. Widespread,
rapid emergence of penicillin resistance among strains of *S. pneumoniae*
is a worldwide concern. The clinical significance of intermediate
penicillin resistance in the management of pneumococcal pneumonia

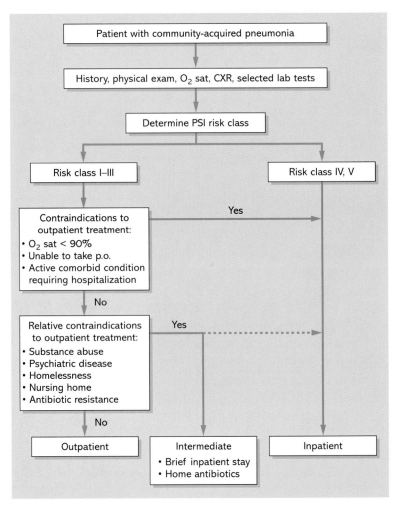

Figure 1.4 Management by risk group for outpatient, intermediate and inpatient care of patients with community-acquired pneumonia. Adapted in part from Halm EA, Fine MJ. Community-acquired pneumonia. In: Wachter RM, Goldman L, Hollander H, eds. *Hospital Medicine*. Philadelphia: Lippincott Williams & Wilkins, 2000.

remains controversial. For high-level penicillin resistance (> 2 µg/mL), vancomycin is the antibiotic of choice. Note that a proportion of these isolates may be multi-drug-resistant to the macrolides, cephalosporins, clindamycin, trimethoprim–sulfamethoxazole and other antibiotics.

TABLE 1.5

Assessment of criteria for severe pneumonia

Factors indicative of severe pneumonia:

- Mechanically ventilated
- Treatment with vasopressors for > 4 h
- Systolic blood pressure < 90 mmHg or diastolic blood pressure < 60 mmHg)
- Urine output < 20 mL/h, or total urine output < 80 mL in 4 h without another cause, or acute renal failure requiring dialysis
- Respiratory rate > 30/min at admission
- Severe respiratory failure defined by a PaO_2/FiO_2 ratio < 250 mmHg
- Chest radiograph showing bilateral involvement or involvement of multiple lobes; an increase in the size of the opacity by 50% or greater within 48 h of admission

Taken from Niederman MS et al. 2001

TABLE 1.6

Guidelines for the treatment of outpatients with CAP

Generally preferred:

- Macrolides*
- Quinolone[†] (3rd or 4th generation)
- Doxycycline

Modifying factors:

- Suspected penicillin resistance: use quinolones[†]
- Suspected aspiration: use ampicillin–sulbactam
- Young adult (17–40 years): use doxycycline
- Older patients or underlying disease: use quinolone[†]

* Azithromycin, clarithromycin, erythromycin
[†] Moxifloxacin, gatifloxacin, levofloxacin
Taken from guidelines published by the Infectious Diseases Society of America (2000),
American Thoracic Society (2001) and British Thoracic Society (2002)

TABLE 1.7

Guidelines for managing inpatients and ICU patients with CAP

General medical ward

Generally preferred:

- β-lactam + macrolide*
- Quinolone (alone)†
- β-lactam + β-lactamase inhibitor

ICU patients with serious pneumonia

Generally preferred if no risk factors:

- Cefotaxime, cefepime or ceftriaxone + macrolide* or quinolone† +/– aminoglycoside
- β-lactam + β-lactamase inhibitor + macrolide* or quinolone† +/– aminoglycoside

Modifying factors:

- *Risk factors for MRSA*: add vancomycin
- *Structural lung disease*: use anti-*Pseudomonas* penicillin, carbapenem or cefepime + macrolide or quinolone + aminoglycoside**
- *Suspected aspiration*: add clindamycin or metronidazole to quinolone or cephalosporin

* Azithromycin, clarithromycin or erythromycin
† Moxifloxacin, levofloxacin or gatifloxacin
** Ampicillin/sulbactam or ticarcillin/clavulanate or piperacillin/tazobactam (for structural disease of the lung, ticarcillin/clavulanate or piperacillin)
Source: Bartlett JG et al. 2000

Use of third- and fourth-generation quinolones, such as gatifloxacin, moxifloxacin or levofloxacin, should be effective. Because of high-level third-generation cephalosporin resistance, caution is advised; these drugs should be considered second-line treatment. In severely ill patients residing in communities where high-level resistance to penicillin is > 5%, adding vancomycin empirically to the initial regimen is recommended. These data emphasize how important it is for clinicians to be aware of the changing patterns of antibiotic resistance in their geographic area.

Assessing clinical response. In most patients there is evidence of clinical improvement in the first 4–48 hours. For patients who improve rapidly on therapy, consideration should be given to an early switch from parenteral to oral therapy, as well as possible discharge from the hospital. The criteria for switching from i.v. to oral therapy, and for earlier discharge, are summarized in Table 1.8.

Although the duration of therapy has not been studied in detail, a total course of 7 to 10 days is probably optimal for most patients. Patients with documented *L. pneumophila* may require 14–21 days of therapy. Patients with underlying lung disease and those who are slow to respond to therapy or have complications may require longer courses.

The differential diagnoses for lack of response or for progression of infection include 'wrong bug' (such as tularemia, *Acinetobacter*, or MRSA), 'wrong drug' (drug-resistant pathogen), wrong diagnosis (noninfectious etiology such as pulmonary embolism) or complication

TABLE 1.8

Criteria for switch from parenteral to oral therapy and hospital discharge

Criteria for switch:

- Stable vital signs for ≥ 24 hours
- Temperature ≤ 37.8° (100°F)
- Spontaneous respiratory rate ≤ 24 breaths/min
- Systolic blood pressure ≥ 90 mmHg
- Normal oxygenation on room air (O_2 sat 90%)
- Able to ingest capsules or liquids
- No evidence of a metastatic infection site

Criteria for discharge

- Conversion to oral antibiotics outlined above
- Able to tolerate oral antibiotics (give first dose in hospital)
- Baseline mental status
- No evidence of comorbid condition needing inpatient care

(metastatic seeding, empyema) (Table 1.9). In such cases, further diagnostic tests and early consultation with a pulmonary or infectious-disease specialist is strongly suggested.

Local complications

Empyema is the most common local complication of pneumococcal pneumonia. A reactive effusion can occur but is trivial; empyema is potentially more serious and is presumably due to bacteria reaching the pleural space via the lymphatics. Clinically, this is signaled by the persistence of fever and leukocytosis after 4–5 days of appropriate antibiotic therapy. Empyema is also suggested by large amounts of pleural fluid evident on the chest radiograph. Ultrasound is often useful

TABLE 1.9

Differential diagnosis of failure to respond or progression

Correct diagnosis	Incorrect diagnosis
Wrong bug	• Congestive heart failure
• Drug-resistant organism	• Embolus
• Other bacterial pathogens	• Neoplasm
• Mycobacteria	• Sarcoidosis
• Nocardia	• Drug reaction
• Fungi	• Hemorrhage
• Viruses	
Wrong drug	
• Error in dose or route	
• Compliance	
Complication	
• Obstruction	
• Superinfection	
• Empyema	
• Abscess	

in determining the site of effusion and identifying the loculae that are typical of empyema (Figure 1.5). Empyema should be drained by repeated needle aspiration or a chest tube; thoracotomy is rarely necessary. Fibrolytic agents, such as urokinase or streptokinase, are being increasingly used to break down loculae.

Lung abscess may be detected radiographically as a fluid level within an area of consolidation on the chest radiograph. This can occur in disease due to *S. pneumoniae* and is classically seen in patients with staphylococcal or *Klebsiella* pneumonia. It can occur in patients with a mixed anaerobic infection, for example, as a result of severe dental infection or in patients with pneumonia secondary to aspiration of vomit, such as vagrants with alcoholism or individuals after epileptic fits or cerebrovascular accidents. Management includes surgical drainage and long-term therapy with β-lactam agents plus an aminoglycoside, or clindamycin plus ciprofloxacin.

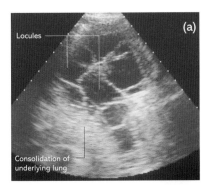

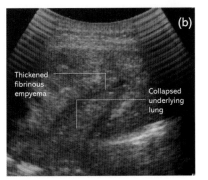

Figure 1.5 Ultrasound images of patients with empyema: (a) note the loculated empyema and the underlying consolidation within lung parenchyma; (b) this patient has thickened, fibrous empyema and a collapsed underlying lung.

Prevention

There are several important long- and short-term targets for prevention of CAP. Clearly, early appropriate antibiotic therapy reduces mortality and morbidity. In addition, in discharge planning, emphasis must be placed on use of vaccines and targeted risk reduction, such as smoking cessation. Data clearly indicate that the use of influenza vaccine decreases healthcare costs, the risk of pneumonia, hospitalization and outpatient visits. Therefore, in the USA it is recommended that all patients with pneumonia should receive yearly influenza vaccine. These patients should be also be vaccinated with the 23-valent pneumococcal polysaccharide vaccine in the hospital or at the patient's initial follow-up visit after discharge. The polysaccharide vaccine is effective for at least 5 years. Revaccination 5 years later is recommended. The use of a new, highly immunogenic polysaccharide–protein conjugate pneumococcal vaccine is likely to have improved efficacy and is currently recommended for use in children and under investigation in adults.

Clinicians should be aware that bacteremic pneumococcal pneumonia may be the initial presenting sign of infection with human immunodeficiency virus, especially in young patients and those with known risk factors for human immunodeficiency virus (HIV) disease. Such patients should be offered HIV testing and counseling.

Long-term prevention of recurrent pneumonia and respiratory tract infections is also of critical importance. Patients who are smoking should be strongly counseled to quit and informed of smoking cessation programs and available strategies to help them with their addiction. Information and educational materials are available on the internet, from government and state health departments and, in the USA, from the Centers for Disease Control and the American Cancer Society and American Lung Association; in the UK, from NHS Direct, ASH or Cancer Research UK. We recommend that all patients have a follow-up appointment to assure compliance with therapy and with risk reduction recommendations and to exclude a complication.

In the USA, the Joint Commission for the Accreditation of Healthcare Organizations (JCAHO) has targeted CAP and will review charts to ensure that appropriate antibiotics defined in the current

Community-acquired pneumonia – Key points

- Pneumococci with high-level resistance to penicillin (> 2 µg/mL) are associated with clinical failure in patients with CAP treated with penicillin.
- Patients admitted from a nursing home or those who have received prior antibiotic therapy are at greater risk for MDR pathogens. However, these strains are usually sensitive to third- and fourth-generation quinolones and all are sensitive to vancomycin.
- Mortality for CAP is associated with high PSI scores, greater severity of disease and inappropriate antibiotic therapy.
- Early antibiotic therapy (< 8 hours from the time of arrival at the hospital) with appropriate initial antibiotics reduces patient mortality.
- Initial antibiotic therapy based on severity of disease has been highlighted in the recent IDSA, ATS and BTS Guidelines. Antibiotic therapy should be reassessed on the basis of culture and response to initial therapy; response should be monitored to identify non-responders and those eligible for early switch from intravenous to oral therapy.
- Effective prevention strategies for CAP include vaccination with pneumococcal or influenza vaccines and smoking cessation.

guidelines were given within 8 hours of entry into the hospital, that blood culture and oxygen concentration were recorded and that a plan for vaccination and for smoking cessation (if applicable) was discussed with the patient.

Hospitals should also consider monitoring the management of pneumonia in their institution and discuss methods to streamline care and improve outcomes. Clearly, the use of the clinical pathway for pneumonia or the routine use of outpatient therapy based on the PSI score, with an earlier switch from parenteral to oral antibiotics and more rapid discharge from the hospital, can markedly reduce hospital costs and improve patient outcomes. Furthermore, overutilization of hospital resources for diagnosis and management should be assessed periodically.

Key references

Niederman MS, Mandell LA, Anzueto A et al. American Thoracic Society Guidelines for the management of adults with community-acquired pneumonia: diagnosis, assessment of severity, antimicrobial therapy and prevention. *Am J Respir Crit Care Med* 2001; 163:1730–54.

BTS Guidelines for the management of community acquired pneumonia in adults. *Thorax* 2001;56(suppl 4): IV1–64.

Bartlett JG, Dowell SF, Mandell LA et al. Practice guidelines for the management of community-acquired pneumonia in adults. Infectious Diseases Society of America. *Clin Infect Dis* 2000;31:347–82.

Fine MJ, Auble TE, Yealy DM et al. A prediction rule to identify low-risk patients with community-acquired pneumonia. *N Engl J Med* 1997;336:243–50.

Marrie TJ, Lau CY, Wheeler SL, Wong CJ et al. A controlled trial of a critical pathway for treatment of community-acquired pneumonia. CAPITAL Study Investigators. Community-Acquired Pneumonia Intervention Trial Assessing Levofloxacin. *JAMA* 2000;283: 749–55.

Hospital-acquired pneumonia (HAP) or nosocomial pneumonia is defined as a new infection of lung parenchyma appearing more than 48 hours after admission to the hospital. HAP is a worldwide problem, a significant cause of patient mortality and morbidity, and a major contributor to increased hospital costs.

Epidemiology

HAP is the second most common nosocomial infection in the United States, but has the highest mortality and morbidity. Most cases of HAP occur outside the ICU, but rates of HAP are highest in mechanically ventilated patients. The use of an endotracheal tube increases the risk of HAP six- to twentyfold, and thus prompt removal when possible is recommended.

Rates of HAP are usually between 5 and 15 cases per 1000 hospital admissions; the incidence density of ventilator-associated pneumonia (VAP) varies from 10 to 25 episodes/1000 ventilator days. Rates vary by the method used for diagnosis, denominators used, and patient population studied. Independent risk factors for HAP include host factors, numbers and virulence of the pathogen, use of medications that alter consciousness, use of invasive devices and host flora (Table 2.1).

Crude mortality rates for ICU patients with HAP are two to ten times higher than for ICU patients without pneumonia. Rates of HAP and VAP are also increased in patients with secondary bacteremia or infection caused by high-risk, MDR pathogens.

Risk factors for mortality in critically ill patients include shock, coma, high APACHE scores, systemic inflammatory response syndrome (SIRS), ultimately and rapidly fatal underlying disease, isolation of the MDR pathogens *Pseudomonas aeruginosa* and *Acinetobacter* spp., bilateral infiltrates on chest x-ray, adult respiratory distress syndrome (ARDS) and respiratory failure. Crude mortality for HAP and VAP ranges from 20% to 50% and attributable mortality, or mortality directly related to the pneumonia, is usually in the 30%s.

TABLE 2.1

Overview of the major independent risk factors for HAP

Host factors:
- Age > 55 yrs
- Obesity
- Hyperglycemia
- Severity of chronic and acute disease
- Presence of chronic lung and cardiac disease
- Presence of organ failure
- Depressed consciousness
- Supine body position
- Poor nutrition
- Alcoholism
- Smoking

Use of invasive devices:
- Intubation and duration of mechanical ventilation
- Nasotracheal tube
- Nasogastric tube
- Parenteral and enteral feeding

Medications:
- Prior antibiotic use
- Use of sedatives, narcotics and neuromuscular blockers
- Histamine type 2 blockers and antacids

Pathogenesis

Aspiration of bacteria from the aerodigestive tract is the most common route of infection (Figure 2.1). Approximately 45% of healthy subjects aspirate during sleep, and aspiration is more frequent in patients with pathologically altered consciousness, abnormal swallowing, depressed gag reflexes, delayed gastric emptying or decreased gastrointestinal motility.

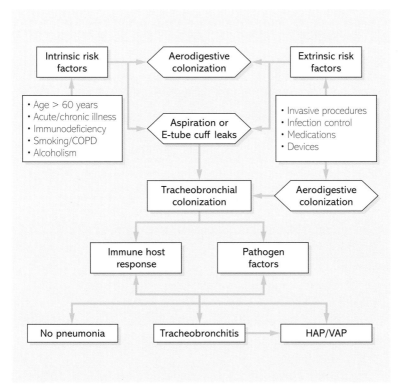

Figure 2.1 Pathogenesis of hospital-acquired or ventilator-associated pneumonia (HAP/VAP). Taken with permission from Fleming et al. 2001.

The development of HAP requires the entry into the lower airway of either a large number of organisms or a smaller number of organisms with greater virulence. For example, enzymes and capsules present in strains of *S. aureus*, or toxins produced by certain strains of *P. aeruginosa*, increase virulence and alter host defenses in the lung.

The pulmonary host defenses constitute a complex system of mechanical, mucosal, humoral and cellular components that protect the host against infection. The dynamic, unique interactions of microorganisms with different host defenses determine if the final outcome is colonization, tracheobronchitis or pneumonia. These patient outcomes are often difficult to characterize because of the wide spectrum of etiologic agents involved, a high rate of mixed infections, and the complexity of host responses.

In the mechanically ventilated patient, local trauma and inflammation from the endotracheal tube and possible leakage of contaminated secretions around the cuff into the upper trachea increase the risk of tracheal colonization, tracheobronchitis and VAP.

Host factors, the types and adherence of bacteria colonizing the pharynx, and the prior exposure to antibiotics may alter colonization and affect pathogenesis. Clearly, hospitalized patients with acute and chronic underlying diseases appear to have higher rates of oropharyngeal colonization with Gram-negative bacilli than normal hosts. Aspiration of bacteria in gastric contents or retrograde colonization of the oropharynx from the stomach may also increase levels of oropharyngeal colonization and the risk HAP and VAP. The stomach is usually sterile at a pH < 2, but log increases in colonization have been noted as gastric acidity is decreased. Increases in colonization from 100 000 to > 1 million bacteria/mL of gastric juice may occur when gastric pH becomes > 3.5 in patients. Advanced age, achlorhydria, various gastrointestinal diseases, malnutrition, and treatment or prophylaxis with antacids and histamine type 2 (H2) blockers may all reduce gastric acidity.

Etiologic agents. Bacteria that commonly cause HAP can be conceptually divided into agents of early- and late-onset disease (Table 2.2). Early HAP occurs during the first four days of the hospital stay and is usually caused by *Streptococcus pneumoniae* and *Haemophilus influenzae*, and sometimes *Moraxella catarrhalis*. By comparison, late-onset pneumonia occurs > 4 days after admission and is more commonly caused by hospital-acquired, aerobic, Gram-negative bacilli, *S. aureus*, *Legionella pneumophila* or rarely *Aspergillus fumigatus*. In 30–50% of patients, HAP is caused by multiple organisms.

Risk factors for colonization with specific types of aerobic Gram-positive cocci and Gram-negative bacilli are summarized in Table 2.3. Anaerobic bacteria have been isolated from about 35% of all cases of nosocomial pneumonia, but are considerably less important in intubated patients and late-onset VAP. *L. pneumophila* occurs episodically, but is more common in hospitals with colonized cooling towers or water supplies.

TABLE 2.2

Spectrum and crude frequency of pathogens associated with HAP classified by time of onset

Pathogen	Onset of pneumonia	Crude frequency
Common pathogens		
Streptococcus pneumoniae	Early	10–20%
Haemophilus influenzae	Early	5–15%
Anaerobic bacteria	Early	10–30%*
Staphylococcus aureus	Early/late	20–30%
Gram-negative bacilli†	Late	30–60%
Legionella pneumophila	Late	0–15%
Uncommon pathogens		
Influenza A and B	Late	< 1%
Respiratory syncytial virus**	Late	0–15%
Aspergillus fumigatus	Late	< 1%
Pneumocystis carinii	Late	< 1%
Mycobacterium tuberculosis	Late	< 1%

* Low in patients with late-onset VAP
† *Escherichia coli, Klebsiella pneumoniae, Enterobacter* spp., *Serratia marcescens, Acinetobacter* spp., *Pseudomonas aeruginosa*
** May cause seasonal epidemics, especially in pediatric patients

Epidemic influenza pneumonia is seasonal and always of concern, while respiratory syncytial virus occurs commonly in pediatric intensive care units. *Candida albicans* often colonizes the respiratory tract, but is an uncommon pathogen except in immunocompromised patients. *A. fumigatus* is also rare, but should be considered if the patient is neutropenic or immunocompromised, or if there is active hospital construction.

Clinical presentation

Clinical evaluation. Symptoms suggesting HAP include fever, cough, purulent sputum production, dyspnea, pleuritic chest pain or change in

TABLE 2.3

Risk factors predisposing to different microbial etiologies in nosocomial pneumonia

Staphylococcus aureus
- Diabetes
- Elderly
- Renal failure
- Recent influenza
- Recent head injury
- Trauma

Pseudomonas aeruginosa
- Malnourishment
- Steroid treatment
- Chronic lung disease
- Prolonged mechanical ventilation
- Prolonged intensive care

Legionella pneumophila
- Immunosuppression
- Steroid treatment
- Contamination of hospital water facilities

Anaerobes
- Recent thoracoabdominal surgery
- Gross aspiration

Viruses (RSV, influenza A, para-influenza, adenovirus)
- Young age (0–5 years)

Haemophilus influenzae
- Chronic lung disease

mental status. Physical examination may reveal a patient appearing ill, with fever, tachycardia and tachypnea progressing to cyanosis and respiratory distress in severe cases. Typical signs of consolidation including coarse crepitations and bronchial breath sounds on auscultation, tactile fremitus and dullness to percussion may be present. Involvement of the pleural space results in signs suggestive of a pleural effusion.

Laboratory data. The initial evaluation of patients with suspected HAP involves confirming the presence of an intrapulmonary parenchymal process and ruling out alternative diagnoses such as atelectasis, pulmonary embolus, or congestive heart failure (Figure 2.2). Computed tomography (CT) may help in diagnosing pneumonia and probable complications such as empyema and lung abscess (Figure 2.3). A false

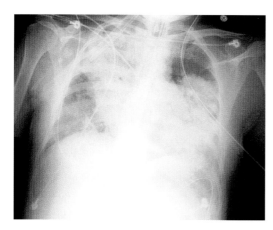

Figure 2.2 Chest x-ray of a patient with HAP/VAP.

Figure 2.3 CT scan of a patient with HAP/VAP.

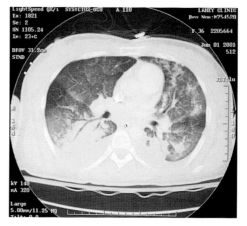

negative chest x-ray is uncommon in HAP but may occur in patients with neutropenia in early HAP. The ability of dehydration to obscure a pulmonary infiltrate on admission or during the first 24 hours after admission is controversial and uncommon.

In patients with a significant parapneumonic effusion, a diagnostic thoracocentesis should be performed to rule out a complicating empyema. Testing for human immunodeficiency virus should be considered for younger patients with pneumococcal pneumonia, particularly if there are any risk factors for HIV disease.

Additional indicators of pneumonia include the quantity or purulence of secretions, increased oxygen requirements, leukocytosis, and a new infiltrate on chest x-ray. Routine laboratory tests recommended for patients with HAP include a complete blood count to assess leukocytosis and anemia, two sets of blood cultures, and sputum for Gram stain, culture or special tests. Positive blood cultures that may identify an infecting organism occur in up to 8–20% of cases and may predict a more complicated course and identify patient groups with a higher mortality.

A properly prepared sputum Gram stain of purulent sputum, examined for cell types and predominant organisms such as pneumococci, staphylococci, anaerobes or nosocomial Gram-negative bacilli, may provide initial clues to the infecting bacteria and important data for correlation with the sputum culture result. Sputum smears having white blood cells without bacteria should raise the suspicion of atypical organisms such as viruses, *Legionella* or mycobacterial species.

Although the sputum culture may have low specificity, especially if the quantity and quality of the sample is poor, it may be useful for identifying antibiotic-resistant organisms. If *Legionella* is suspected, sputum should be cultured on appropriate media and examined by direct fluorescent antibody (DFA) or samples sent for testing for *Legionella* serotype 1 urinary antigen.

Oxygenation should be assessed initially by pulse oximetry and an arterial blood gas determination should be considered in critically ill patients and those with an oxygen saturation of less than 92%. Chemistry profiles, including electrolytes to screen for hyponatremia, acidosis screening, and liver and kidney function tests (elevated blood urea nitrogen, BUN) to determine other organ dysfunction should be performed routinely at the time of diagnosis and as needed thereafter.

Clinical diagnosis of ventilator-associated pneumonia, using the criteria of a new infiltrate on chest x-ray in mechanically ventilated patients with fever, sputum production or leukocytosis, is sensitive but not specific, leading to overdiagnosis and unnecessary antibiotic treatment.

Some clinical investigators have used the clinical pulmonary infection score (CPIS) to assist in the diagnosis of HAP and VAP. The CPIS gives a number of points for patient body temperature, leukocyte count, presence of purulent secretions, levels of oxygenation, infiltrates on chest x-ray and the isolation of pathogens on bacterial culture

(Table 2.4). The CPIS score varies from 0 to 12 points; scores > 6 correlated well with the bronchoscopic diagnosis of pneumonia, and patients with a score < 6 have a lower likelihood of HAP.

Bronchoscopy or 'blind' BAL/PSB for VAP. Recent data from a multicenter study in France suggested that patients with VAP who were diagnosed by bronchoscopy with bronchoalveolar lavage (BAL) and/or protected specimen brush (PSB) had significantly decreased length of stay, mortality and antibiotic use compared with patients whose diagnosis was made by clinical criteria alone. Unfortunately, the

TABLE 2.4

Clinical pulmonary infection score (CPIS)* used for the diagnosis of VAP

Criterion	Value	Points
Temperature (°C)	36.5–38.4	0
	38.5–39.0	1
	< 36.5 or > 39.0	2
Blood leukocytes	4000–11 000	0
(mm^{-3})	< 4000 or > 11 000	1
	≥ 500 band forms	+1
Tracheal secretions	< 14 times secretions suctioned / 24 h	0
	≥ 14 times secretions suctioned / 24 h	1
	purulent secretions	+1
Oxygenation:	>240 or ARDS	0
PaO_2/FiO_2 (mmHg)	< 240 and no evidence of ARDS	2
Pulmonary	No infiltrate	0
radiography	Diffused (or patchy) infiltrate	1
	Localized infiltrate	2
Culture and Gram stain	No pathogenic bacteria cultured (0/+)	0
of tracheal aspirate	Pathogenic bacteria cultured (+/++/+++)	1
(semiquantitative:	Pathogenic bacteria on Gram stain (>+)	+1
0/+/++/+++)		

* Total CPIS points ≥ 6 consistent with diagnosis of VAP.
Adapted from Pugin et al. 1991.
PaO_2, arterial oxygen pressure; FiO_2, inspiratory oxygen concentration

availability of bronchoscopy is limited and resources in the microbiology laboratory are limited in many hospitals. Care is advised in collecting and interpreting these data in patents who have received new antibiotics in the previous 24–48 hours and when interpreting mixed infections (those due to anaerobes and *Candida* spp.).

Bronchoscopy with BAL or PSB may also be useful for severely ill patients, those suspected of harboring unusual pathogens or those who do not respond to empiric antibiotic therapy.

The use of 'blind' BAL and quantitative bacteriology has also improved the specificity of the diagnosis of VAP. This technique has greater availability and application for the diagnosis of VAP, but requires appropriate laboratory support.

Quantitative endotracheal aspirates (QEA) for VAP. If no invasive techniques are to be used on intubated patients with suspected HAP, endotracheal aspirate should be obtained for Gram stain and quantitative culture. Quantitative endotracheal aspirates having 10^5 or 10^6 organisms/mL correlate well with 10^4 organisms/mL by BAL or 10^3 organisms/mL for PSB samples. The use of QEA along with the clinical diagnosis is probably superior to clinical diagnosis alone and provides similar results and outcomes to those obtained by bronchoscopy with BAL and PSB.

Management

The 1995 American Thoracic Society's Guideline for the Management of HAP provides the principles for initial antibiotic therapy. Initial antibiotic therapy should be based on the severity of disease, whether onset is early or late, and specific risk factors associated with nosocomial pathogens (Figure 2.4, Tables 2.3, 2.5 and 2.6).

Intravenous antibiotics, which are often empiric, should be initiated as soon as possible after appropriate blood and sputum cultures are obtained to limit progression of disease and associated complications (Tables 2.5 and 2.6). In choosing the optimal empiric intravenous antibiotic regimen, consideration should be given to the resistance patterns of prevalent, endemic nosocomial pathogens, exposure to prior antibiotics, or to prior hospitalization in chronic care facilities.

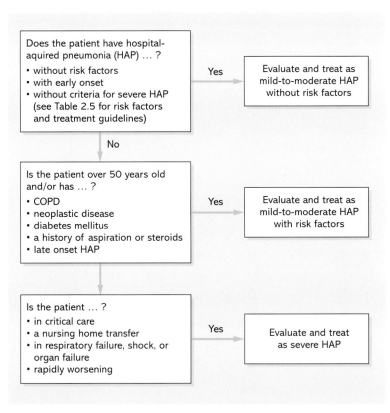

Figure 2.4 Decision tree for initial antibiotic therapy based on the severity of disease and risk factors for specific etiologic agents. Taken from Craven DE et al. 2000.

Mild-to-moderate HAP. Patients with mild-to-moderate disease and without risk factors are usually infected with one of the 'core' pathogens and should be treated with one or more of the intravenous antibiotics summarized in Tables 2.5 and 2.6. Patients with risk factors for anaerobes, atypical pathogens such as *Legionella* or methicillin-resistant *S. aureus* (MRSA) may need additional antibiotics. In contrast to the β-lactams, quinolones and macrolides such as azithromycin have activity against atypical pathogens such as *Mycoplasma pneumoniae*, *Chlamydia pneumoniae* and against *L. pneumophila*. Note that fourth-generation quinolones, such as gatifloxacin, have better anaerobic activity than levofloxacin or ciprofloxacin.

TABLE 2.5

Summary of clinical setting, organisms, and empiric treatment of HAP based on severity of disease (adapted in part from the American Thoracic Society Guidelines)

Mild or moderate HAP

No risk factors	Core organisms
No unusual risk factors Early onset	S. pneumoniae, H. influenzae, S. aureus, E. coli, Klebsiella Enterobacter spp. Serratia spp.

With risk factors	Other pathogens
Recent abdominal surgery Witnessed aspiration	Core organisms + anaerobes
High-dose steroids	L. pneumophila
Prior hospitalization ICU stay Steroids Prior antibiotics Chronic lung disease	P. aeruginosa and MRSA

Severe HAP

Clinical setting	
ICU Nursing home Prior antibiotics Respiratory failure Progressive pneumonia Sepsis, shock Organ failure	Core organisms + P. aeruginosa + Legionella pneumophila + MRSA

* MRSA, methicillin-resistant S. aureus

Initial antibiotics

2nd- or 3rd-generation cephalosporin
OR
3rd- or 4th-generation quinolone
OR
β-lactam + β-lactamase inhibitor

Initial antibiotics

2nd- or 3rd-generation cephalosporin + clindamycin
OR
4th-generation quinolone alone
OR
β-lactam + β-lactamase inhibitor

Use macrolide or quinolone

Treat as severe HAP

Initial antibiotics

3rd- or 4th-generation antipseudomonal cephalosporin + quinolone
± vancomycin
OR
3rd- or 4th-generation antipseudomonal cephalosporin + macrolide
± vancomycin ± aminoglycoside
OR
carbapenem + quinolone ± vancomycin

Severe pneumonia. For patients with severe pneumonia, broad-spectrum, combination antibiotic coverage should be prescribed to sufficiently cover all potential bacterial pathogens, including *L. pneumophila*, *P. aeruginosa*, other antibiotic-resistant nosocomial Gram-negative bacilli, and MRSA (Tables 2.5 and 2.6). Although the specific antibiotic regimen should be based on the prevalent endemic pathogens in the hospital or ICU, the use of a third- or fourth-generation cephalosporin with activity against *P. aeruginosa*, such as ceftazidime or cefepime, or a broad-spectrum β-lactam such as imipenem or meropenem is suggested, in combination with a quinolone, such as ciprofloxacin, levofloxacin or gatifloxacin. Aminoglycosides may be considered for initial coverage against MDR Gram-negative bacilli, but difficulties in dosing to achieve sufficient serum levels and poor penetration into inflamed lung tissues are of concern, and side-effects such as nephrotoxicity and ototoxicity should limit their use if other effective antibiotics are effective.

The optimal duration of therapy for HAP is unknown, but antibiotics are generally given for 10 to 14 days. Shorter courses of antibiotics may be used in early-onset VAP than in late-onset. Data from a randomized clinical trial indicated that patients with a CPIS score < 6 (a low likelihood of HAP, Table 2.4) can be safely treated for 3 days with ciprofloxacin, and if the CPIS score remains < 6 at day 3, antibiotics can be stopped. These data support the use of shorter courses and oral antibiotics in low-risk patients, but independent verification of these results is needed.

Patients with more severe underlying disease, impaired immune systems, or infection with more antibiotic-resistant organisms often receive longer courses of antibiotics. Patients with complications such as lung abscess or empyema may require 4 to 8 weeks of antibiotic treatment along with other interventions, which are discussed in a later section. If there is a rapid response to antibiotic therapy, the duration of therapy for some pathogens may be shortened. After the patient's condition stabilizes, the prescribed course may be completed in step-down facilities or at home. Once the pathogen is identified and the in vitro susceptibility confirmed, if the patient is responding to therapy and there are no contraindications, oral antibiotics may be considered

TABLE 2.6

Selected antimicrobials used for intravenous treatment of HAP in adults

Antibiotic	Limitations	Comments
Cephalosporins: Cefuroxime (2nd) Ceftriaxone (3rd) Ceftazidime (3rd) Cefepime (4th)	No coverage for atypical pathogens, MRSA; limited for anaerobes	3rd and 4th generation have better *P. aeruginosa* activity
β-lactam + β-lactamase inhibitors: Piperacillin + tazobactam Ticarcillin + clavulanic acid	No coverage for atypical pathogens	Add macrolide or quinolone for atypical pathogens
Carbapenems: Imipenem Meropenem	No coverage for atypical pathogens	Add macrolide or quinolone for atypical pathogens
Quinolones: Ciprofloxacin (2nd) Levofloxacin (3rd) Gatifloxacin, moxifloxacin (4th)	2nd generation limited for pneumococci, anaerobes	3rd & 4th generation good for resistant pneumococci; 4th gives better anaerobe coverage
Macrolides: Azithromycin Erythromycin	Limited activity against nosocomial pathogens	Use as additional coverage for atypical pathogens
Clindamycin	MRSA, GNB	Excellent against anaerobes and sensitive *S. aureus*
Aminoglycosides: Gentamicin Tobramycin Amikacin	May penetrate poorly into infected lung tissue; no anaerobe or Gram-positive activity	Other antibiotics for GNB may be better and have less toxicity; good *P. aeruginosa* coverage
Vancomycin	No Gram-negative or atypical coverage	Useful to cover MRSA
Linezolid	No Gram-negative or atypical coverage	Excellent coverage for MRSA and VRE

GNB, Gram-negative bacteria; VRE, vancomycin-resistant enterococci; MRSA, methicillin-resistant *S. aureus*

for the completion of the course of therapy. Currently there are no data to support the use of adjuvant therapies such as granulocyte colony stimulating factor or cytokines in patients with VAP. However, recent data from patients with ARDS suggest that steroids are beneficial.

Response to therapy. Like the initial diagnostic evaluation, assessment of clinical response involves ongoing monitoring of the patient's fever, sputum production, oxygenation, leukocytosis, radiographic infiltrates and other relevant laboratory results. Although the course of HAP may vary, signs of clinical response may occur within 12 to 24 hours, but should be evident 48 to 72 hours after therapy is initiated. Antibiotic therapy can be streamlined at 48 hours when culture and sensitivity data are available.

The usual duration of therapy is 10 to 14 days, but patients with MDR organisms or complications or who have a slow response to antibiotics may need longer therapy. Shorter courses of therapy may be possible for patients with mild to moderate disease who respond quickly to initial therapy.

Once the patient is responding, evaluation for switch from i.v. to oral therapy should begin along with discharge planning, follow-up and use of the appropriate long-term prophylaxis measures discussed below.

Lack of response to therapy, defined as either failure to improve or deterioration, may be due either to the incorrect initial diagnosis of pneumonia, wrong organism or inappropriate antibiotic therapy (Table 2.7). In addition to the direct consequences of HAP, complications may also result from the necessary interventions and treatment. These include *Clostridium difficile* colitis, central venous catheter infections, drug reactions or toxicity, venous thromboembolism and respiratory tract superinfection, seen most frequently in intubated patients. These complications may present as a failure to respond to antibiotic therapy, and need to be considered in the evaluation of the poorly responding patient.

Prophylaxis

Strategies for prevention of HAP can be targeted at host factors, medications and devices that facilitate patient colonization, aspiration, and the environment. Measures for infection control are aimed at preventing cross-infection or colonization with pathogens from other patients and staff and at removal of unnecessary invasive devices or respiratory therapy equipment that may increase the risk of HAP.

Adherence to proper infection control practices, including effective handwashing and the proper use of respiratory and barrier precautions, minimizes cross-infection and spread of MDR Gram-negative bacilli and MRSA. The use of a bedside, alcohol-based hand disinfectant in the ICU increases compliance and decreases rates of nosocomial infection. Patient and staff education and the use of a 'multidisciplinary

TABLE 2.7

Differential diagnosis of patients who fail to respond or who deteriorate following initial therapy

Correct initial diagnosis	Incorrect initial diagnosis
Wrong bug	• Atelectasis
• Bacterial/*Legionella*/mycobacteria	• Neoplasm
• Viral	• Pulmonary embolism
• Fungal/*Pneumocystis carinii*	• Congestive heart failure
	• Acute respiratory distress syndrome
Wrong drug	• Pulmonary hemorrhage
• MRSA	• Pulmonary contusion
• MDR Gram-negative*	• Chemical pneumonitis
Complication	
• Empyema	
• Lung abscess	
• *Clostridium difficile* colitis	
• Central line infection	
• Drug fever	

* Common examples of MDR Gram-negatives include *Pseudomonas aeruginosa, Acinetobacter baumannii, Klebsiella* spp.
Modified from Craven DE et al. Nosocomial pneumonia. In: Wachter RM, Goldman L, Hollander H, eds. *Hospital Medicine*. Philadelphia: Lippincott Williams & Wilkins, 2000:496

team approach' to prophylaxis of nosocomial infections is recommended.

Recommendations are available from evidence-based guidelines from the Centers for Disease Control/Hospital Infection Control Practices Committee (CDC/HICPAC). The 1994 Guideline for the Prevention of Nosocomial Pneumonia will soon be updated, and more recent evidence-based recommendations for prevention of VAP have been published by Kollef (Figure 2.5).

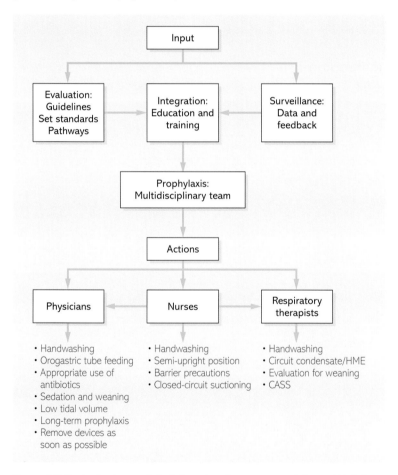

Figure 2.5 Strategies for prophylaxis based on the recommendations of Kollef et al. 1999. CASS, continuous aspiration of subglottic secretions; HME, heat and moisture exchanger. Taken with permission from Fleming CA et al. 2001.

Host factors, such as advanced age, smoking, recent surgery, and underlying diseases significantly increase the risk of pneumonia and colonization of the upper airway. Targets for long-term prophylaxis include smoking cessation and use of pneumococcal and influenza vaccinations in high-risk populations.

Aspiration and gastric reflux are common in hospitalized patients who are elderly, on sedatives or receiving tube feedings. The simple and cost-free practice of maintaining the patient's trunk in a position at least 30 degrees above the horizontal has been associated with a decreased risk of pneumonia. Incentive spirometry and early ambulation may be particularly effective in preventing pneumonia and atelectasis in post-operative patients and those with chronic obstructive pulmonary disease (COPD). Recent data also suggest that tight control of hyper-glycemia in surgical ICU patients will decrease infection and the use of mechanical ventilation and improve patient outcomes. Finally, the risks associated with immobility can be lessened by the use of lateral rotation beds or by assisting the patient with regular position changes or, when possible, early ambulation. Clearly, use of oral rather than nasogastric tubes is recommended, as is removal of all invasive devices.

Prudent use of antimicrobials, especially in the ICU, may reduce emergence of MDR nosocomial pathogens. Cycling or rotating the standard groups of antibiotics used for empiric therapy of infections such as pneumonia has also been efficacious in some hospitals.

Selective decontamination of the digestive tract, in which combinations of antibiotics are applied to the oropharynx and stomach, with and without systemic antibiotics, for prophylaxis against nosocomial pneumonia, may be effective in selected patients or for the eradication of a virulent MDR nosocomial pathogen. These promising results have to be weighed against the risk of long-term selection for MDR organisms.

Sedatives have been associated with an increased risk of aspiration or colonization, and may delay weaning from mechanical ventilation, and should therefore be used judiciously. Similarly, prophylaxis of stress bleeding should be used selectively in high-risk ICU patients. If stress-bleeding prophylaxis is indicated, sucralfate has been associated with a lower risk of late-onset VAP than antacids or histamine type 2 blockers,

Hospital-acquired pneumonia – Key points

- The pathogenesis of HAP/VAP is most commonly related to prior bacterial colonization of the oral pharynx.
- Early-onset HAP or VAP usually occurs in the first 4 days of hospitalization or intubation. These patients are less likely to have antibiotic-resistant organisms and carry a better prognosis than patients with late-onset disease.
- Patients who have received prior antibiotic therapy, those who have been previously hospitalized and ICU patients are more likely to be infected with MDR pathogens.
- Patients hospitalized in the ICU are at greater risk of infections due to pathogens that are endemic to that unit. Agents causing HAP or VAP vary by ICU and geographic region. These data are important in planning initial antibiotic therapy.
- QEA, BAL and PSB increase the specificity of VAP diagnosis. Invasive diagnostic techniques are associated with decreased mortality and better use of antibiotics.
- HAP patients with a CPIS score ≤ 6 at diagnosis may respond to short courses of monotherapy with a quinolone.
- Early appropriate antibiotic therapy improves outcomes in patients with VAP. ATS guidelines suggest empiric choices for initial antimicrobial therapy. When cultures are available, regimens may be streamlined.
- The use of good infection control practices, maintaining patients in the supine position, and limiting exposure to invasive devices such as endotracheal tubes and nasogastric tubes have been suggested to prevent VAP.

but may be less effective in preventing clinically significant bleeding than histamine type 2 blockers.

The use of non-invasive ventilation (NIV) in selected patients has substantially reduced the risk of VAP, antibiotic use and hospital costs, and improved patient outcome. Contaminated devices such as respirometers, ambu bags, temperature sensors, medication nebulizers and bronchoscopes have been associated with an increased risk of pneumonia that can be minimized by proper cleaning and disinfection between patients, and by appropriate use of these devices and, in some cases, expeditious discontinuation. The use of continuous aspiration of subglottic secretions that pool above the endotracheal tube and maintenance of adequate endotracheal cuff pressure will reduce the risk of early-onset VAP. Ventilator tubing need not be changed, and reflux of ventilator tubing condensate into the patient's respiratory tract can be minimized by the use of heat and moisture exchangers. In order to manage secretions optimally and to maintain oxygenation of the patient, closed suctioning systems should be used.

The use of enteral feeding has a lower risk of HAP than parenteral feeding. The risk of aspiration associated with tube feedings may be reduced by verifying tube placement, using continuous as opposed to bolus feedings, properly managing residuals and considering jejunal tube feedings. The use of oral rather than nasogastric and nasotracheal tubes in mechanically ventilated patients may prevent HAP and hospital-acquired sinusitis.

Some of the most effective prevention strategies are widely available, inexpensive and non-invasive, but underutilized for the prevention of HAP. The complexity of risk factors and the spectrum of effective prevention strategies demand the establishment of a team that includes intensivists, nurses, a respiratory therapist and a pharmacist as well as infection control personnel to monitor resistant pathogens and clusters of unusual organisms and to feed back rates of HAP.

Research to delineate the most effective and feasible prevention strategies for HAP has been compromised by insufficient funding and lack of adequate multicenter studies to increase the power and generalizability of results. Unfortunately, many effective strategies for prevention have not been widely disseminated or implemented in hospitals worldwide.

Key references

American Thoracic Society. Hospital-acquired pneumonia in adults: diagnosis, assessment of severity, initial antibiotic therapy and prevention strategies: a consensus statement, November 1995. *Am J Respir Crit Care Med* 1996;153: 1711–25.

Chastre J, Fagon JY. Ventilator-associated pneumonia. *Am J Respir Crit Care Med* 2002;165:867–903.

Fagon JY, Chastre J, Wolff M et al. Invasive and non-invasive strategies for the management of suspected ventilator-associated pneumonia: a randomized trial. *Ann Intern Med* 2000;132:621–30.

Fleming CA, Balaguera HU, Craven DE. Risk factors for nosocomial pneumonia. Focus on prophylaxis. *Med Clin North Am* 2001;85: 1545–63.

Kollef MH. The prevention of ventilator-associated pneumonia. *N Engl J Med* 1999;340:627–34.

Pugin J, Auckenthaler R, Mili N et al. Diagnosis of ventilator-associated pneumonia by bacteriologic analysis of bronchoscopic and nonbronchoscopic "blind" bronchoalveolar lavage fluid. *Am Rev Respir Dis* 1991;143:1121–9.

Singh N, Rogers P, Atwood CW et al. Short course empiric antibiotic therapy for patients with pulmonary infiltrates in the intensive care unit: a proposed solution for indiscriminate antibiotic prescription. *Am J Respir Crit Care Med* 2001;162:505–11.

Tablan OC, Anderson LJ, Arden NH et al. Guideline for prevention of nosocomial pneumonia. The Hospital Infection Control Practices Advisory Committee, Centers for Disease Control and Prevention. *Infect Control Hosp Epidemiol* 1994;15:587–627. Also in: *Am J Infect Control* 1994;22:247–92.

Chronic obstructive pulmonary disease (COPD) is characterized by airflow obstruction due to chronic bronchitis or emphysema; this is defined as a ratio of forced expiratory volume in 1 second to forced vital capacity (FEV_1:FVC) of less than 70%. The decline in FEV_1 with advancing age is much greater in patients with COPD than in normal individuals, and is particularly rapid in those patients who continue to smoke (Figure 3.1). Infective exacerbations are also associated with an acute decline in FEV_1. Although infection is the most common cause of death in patients with COPD, it is unclear whether infective exacerbations lead to an accelerated loss of lung function during the natural history of chronic bronchitis.

Epidemiology

In contrast to statistics for heart disease and cerebrovascular disease, the incidence and prevalence of COPD are increasing. In the USA,

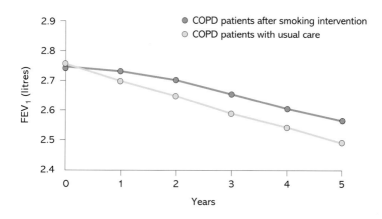

Figure 3.1 The accelerated decline in FEV_1 in individuals with COPD is greatest in those who continue to smoke. Data from Anthonisen et al. 1994.

COPD is the fourth leading cause of death, affecting 14% of adult men and 8% of adult women; UK figures are similar. Infective exacerbations of COPD are common during the winter months and occur, on average, three times per year.

COPD has a significant economic impact. In the UK, chronic bronchitis is associated with a loss of 28 million working days/year. In addition to this, COPD accounts for a large proportion of the £42 million ($61 million) spent on antibiotic prescriptions for lower respiratory tract infections every year in the UK.

Pathology

The underlying pathology of stable COPD is airway remodeling as a consequence of chronic narrowing of the airways. In emphysema, the chronic airflow limitation is due to destruction of the alveolar structures, while in chronic bronchitis, it is due to chronic inflammation secondary to mucous-gland hypertrophy and hyperplasia, and peribronchial fibrosis.

In infective exacerbations of COPD, purulent sputum most commonly yields:

- *H. influenzae*
- *S. pneumoniae*
- *Moraxella catarrhalis*.

Indeed, these organisms are present in many patients between exacerbations, and their number simply increases during the infective episode. In most cases, the initiating factor of an infective exacerbation is unknown, but viral and *Mycoplasma* infections are responsible for up to one third of the acute exacerbations of COPD; the viruses most commonly identified include influenza A, para-influenza virus, coronavirus and rhinovirus.

H. influenzae has an affinity for airway epithelium and attaches to the damaged airway mucosa of patients with COPD (Figure 3.2). It adheres to mucus via pili, and to galactoside sequences on the epithelial cells. Soluble products of *H. influenzae* have been shown to reduce ciliary beat frequency and mucociliary clearance. In patients with more severe disease, Gram-negative bacilli (including *P. aeruginosa*) and *S. aureus* can be recovered from purulent sputum.

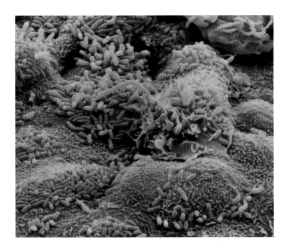

Figure 3.2 Scanning electron micrograph of human airway mucosa showing adherence of *H. influenzae* to the surface epithelial cells (image RC Read and A Brain).

Clinical features

Patients with COPD usually present as a result of an infective exacerbation of the disease, and usually have one or more of the following symptoms:

- increased dyspnea
- increased sputum volume
- increased sputum purulence.

Between exacerbations, patients have exercise limitation as a result of their airways obstruction. This can be staged according to the FEV_1 (Table 3.1).

Investigations

The diagnosis is usually clinically obvious, but investigations necessary in severely ill patients include:

- chest radiograph
- biochemical tests
- hematology
- formal blood gas analysis
- measurement of peak expiratory flow (PEF) and formal spirometry
- sputum culture
- blood culture.

Culture of sputum is of doubtful value in some patients, because it is likely to be contaminated by pathogens that are also present in

TABLE 3.1

Staging of chronic obstructive pulmonary disease

FEV_1 % predicted value	Degree	Stage
> 50	Moderate	I
35–49	Severe	II
< 35	Very severe	III

oropharyngeal secretions. It is therefore important to ensure that only purulent sputum is obtained.

Prognostic indicators

Factors associated with increased morbidity and mortality include:
- decreased lung function (FEV_1 < 1.0 liter)
- blood gas changes – worsening hypercapnia (especially when cardiac disease is present)
- comorbid conditions
- frequent exacerbations
- mucus hypersecretion
- continued smoking
- malnutrition
- treatment with corticosteroids
- increasing age (> 70 years).

Management of COPD

The general management of patients with COPD between infective exacerbations includes:
- encouragement to stop smoking
- respiratory rehabilitation (physiological training: graded physical exercises and breathing exercises)
- long-term oxygen therapy
- drug treatment.

Drug treatment. A stepwise pharmacological management program for COPD has been suggested by Celli.

- Intermittent symptoms should be treated with beta-agonists as required.
- Mild persistent symptoms should be treated with ipratropium plus beta-agonists as required.
- Severe persistent symptoms should be treated with a combination of ipratropium, beta-agonists and theophylline as required; theophylline should be monitored.
- A COPD crisis should be treated with ipratropium and beta-agonists as required, together with a trial of corticosteroids.

Antibiotic therapy. The effect of antibiotics on the outcome of exacerbations in COPD has been assessed in a number of trials. In general, these have shown a small benefit in this heterogeneous population (Table 3.2). The systematic review by Saint et al. (1995) of 1101 patients with acute exacerbations demonstrated a significant, although small, positive effect of antibiotics compared with placebo in terms of simple clinical evidence of improvement and peak expiratory flow rate.

Anthonisen et al. demonstrated that when patients were stratified according to the severity of their exacerbations, there was a clear improvement in clinical outcome with antibiotic therapy in those with the most severe illness (those with at least two out of three of increased dyspnea, sputum volume and sputum purulence). In view of this, Wilson has suggested a simple classification system for the use of antibiotic therapy in COPD that takes into account the baseline clinical status, prognostic markers and likely pathogens (Table 3.3). Simple antibiotic therapy (e.g. an oral aminopenicillin) is recommended for patients with uncomplicated illness, but patients who are older, with poor underlying lung function (FEV_1 ≤ 50% predicted) or comorbid illness, are more likely to have had recurrent courses of antimicrobials and be colonized by resistant organisms. Therefore, in this group, treatment with relatively sophisticated antimicrobials, including amoxicillin–clavulanic acid, ciprofloxacin, second- or third-generation cephalosporins or modern macrolides, is indicated in order to ensure adequate eradication of *H. influenzae*.

TABLE 3.2

Results of trials to assess the effect of antibiotics on the outcome of exacerbations in chronic obstructive pulmonary disease

Source	Setting	Total n patients	Treatment
Elmes et al. 1957	Outpatient	130	Oxytetracycline
Fear and Edwards 1962	Outpatient	119	Oxytetracycline
Pines et al. 1972	Inpatient	149	Tetracycline
Anthonisen et al. 1987	Outpatient	310	Trimethoprim– sulfamethoxazole, amoxicillin, doxycycline
Jorgensen et al. 1992	Outpatient	262	Amoxicillin

PEF, peak expiratory flow
Adapted from Saint et al. 1995

TABLE 3.3

Empiric classifications and suggested therapy for patients with chronic bronchitis

Baseline clinical status	Presenting clinical features
Acute tracheobronchitis	No underlying structural disease
Simple chronic bronchitis	$FEV_1 > 50\%$ Increased sputum volume and purulence
Complicated chronic bronchitis	$FEV_1 < 50\%$ Advanced age ≥ 4 exacerbations/year Significant comorbid disease
Chronic bronchial suppuration (bronchiectasis)	Stage III + continuous purulent sputum production

Main outcome measure	Effect on outcome
Days of illness	Small reduction compared with placebo
Overall score by physician	Moderate improvement compared with placebo
Overall score by physician / change in PEF	Moderate improvement compared with placebo
Days of illness / change in PEF	Moderate benefit in patients with most severe illness only
Overall score by physician / change in PEF	Minimal effect compared with placebo

Pathogens	Suggested antibiotic therapy
Usually viral	None
H. influenzae, Moraxella catarrhalis, S. pneumoniae (possible β-lactam resistance)	Either none, or simple β-lactam therapy
H. influenzae, Moraxella catarrhalis, S. pneumoniae (resistance to β-lactams common)	Amoxicillin–clavulanic acid, quinolone, second- or third-generation cephalosporins, modern macrolide
As with complicated chronic bronchitis + Enterobacteriaceae, P. aeruginosa	High-dose aminopenicillin, high-dose second- or third-generation cephalosporin, high-dose quinolone

Hospitalization is necessary for patients with an acute exacerbation of COPD, characterized by increased dyspnea, cough and sputum production, who have:

- failed to respond to outpatient management
- acute immobility
- inability to eat or sleep due to dyspnea
- high-risk comorbid conditions (e.g. pneumonia, heart failure, cor pulmonale)
- new or worsening hypercapnia or hypoxemia.

Patients who are severely ill may require assisted ventilation including nasal continuous positive airway pressure to support gas exchange. Intubation should not be withheld from patients who have not been ventilated before, because their prognosis is relatively good.

Infective exacerbation of COPD – Key points

- Antibiotic therapy is warranted in patients with severe exacerbations of COPD.
- The presence of comorbidities and other factors influence the type of antibiotic therapy.
- Smoking cessation is imperative.

Key references

Anthonisen NR, Connett JE, Kiley JP et al. Effects of smoking intervention and the use of an inhaled anticholinergic bronchodilator on the rate of decline of FEV_1. The Lung Health Study. *JAMA* 1994;272: 1497–505.

Anthonisen NR, Manfreda J, Warren CP et al. Antibiotic therapy in exacerbations of chronic obstructive pulmonary disease. *Ann Intern Med* 1987;106:196–204.

Celli BR. Pulmonary rehabilitation in patients with COPD. *Am J Respir Crit Care Med* 1995;152:861–4.

Pines A, Khaja G, Greenfield JS et al. A double-blind comparison of slow-release tetracycline and tetracycline hydrochloride in purulent exacerbations of chronic bronchitis. *Br J Clin Pract* 1972;26:475–6.

Jorgensen AF, Coolidge J, Pedersen PA et al. Amoxicillin in treatment of acute uncomplicated exacerbations of chronic bronchitis. A double-blind, placebo-controlled multicentre study in general practice. *Scand J Prim Health Care* 1992;10:7–11.

Saint S, Bent S, Vittinghoff E, Grady D. Antibiotics in chronic obstructive pulmonary disease exacerbations: a meta-analysis. *JAMA* 1995;273: 957–60.

Pulmonary tuberculosis, always prevalent in developing countries, has now re-emerged as a significant problem in many developed countries. This is a reversal of the decline in the incidence of the disease, and the consequent reduction in mortality, seen between the 1940s and the 1970s. The positive influence of improvements in social welfare and the development of effective antituberculous agents has been counteracted by problems of AIDS, urban decline and overcrowding, immigration and the specter of multi-drug-resistant *Mycobacterium tuberculosis*.

Epidemiology

Approximately one third of the world's population – 1.7 billion people – have been infected by *M. tuberculosis* at some time. Of the 100 million people who become infected every year, about 10% will develop tuberculosis (TB) and many will die as a result. In 1994, approximately 3 million people (a third of whom were children) died of TB. Furthermore, the annual incidence of TB in most developed countries is rising; figures published by the WHO showed a rise of 5–30% between 1989 and 1992. However, in the USA there has been a sharp reduction in the number of reported cases thanks to comprehensive improvement of control activities.

The worldwide distribution of cases of TB is shown in Figure 4.1. The prevalence of HIV is a significant epidemiological factor in areas with a high incidence of TB. In sub-Saharan Africa, almost 50% of individuals in the age group most susceptible to HIV infection (15–45 years) are infected with *M. tuberculosis*, compared with about 12% in the USA and Western Europe.

Pathogenesis

The *Mycobacterium tuberculosis* complex is dominated by two closely related species – *M. tuberculosis* and *M. bovis*. *M. tuberculosis* is mainly transmitted by droplet spread from coughing patients. *M. bovis* remains a problem in areas where agricultural control measures have not been instituted, and is spread to farm workers by diseased cattle or to urban dwellers in unpasteurized milk.

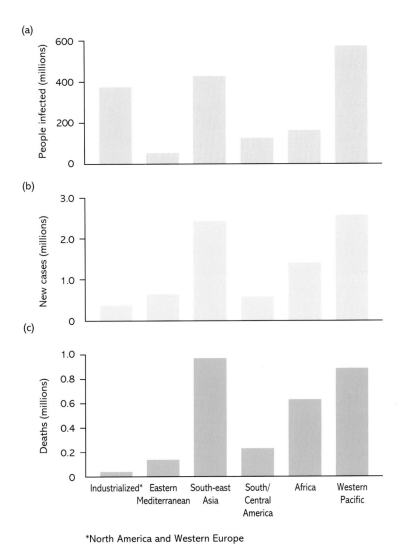

Figure 4.1 Estimated worldwide (a) prevalence, (b) incidence and (c) mortality of tuberculosis in 1991. Data from Kochi A. The global tuberculosis situation and the new control strategy of the WHO. *Tubercle* 1991;72:1–6.

Transmission occurs almost exclusively via patients whose sputum is smear-positive (i.e. contains ≥ 5000 bacilli/mL). Approximately 10% of non-immunocompromised individuals who become infected eventually develop overt disease. Of these, 50% will develop 'primary disease' (i.e. within 5 years of infection), while the other 50% will develop 'post-primary disease'. Once inhaled, *M. tuberculosis* is taken up by macrophages, but normal lung macrophages are incapable of killing *M. tuberculosis* and require activation by CD4+ cells via interferon (IFN)-γ. Activated macrophages aggregate to form characteristic granulomas, which together with a lymphocytic infiltrate produce IFN-γ and other cytokines, including tumor necrosis factor (TNF). Tubercle bacilli are destroyed by a combination of intracellular killing and the anoxia within the middle of the granuloma that results from necrosis.

Approximately 95% of primarily infected individuals kill tubercle bacilli by this mechanism, though some bacilli may survive for years in a dormant state. If bacilli are not effectively killed locally, they are transported to regional lymph nodes and are taken up by dendritic cells for antigen presentation. Other bacilli disseminate throughout the body, including the CNS.

Clinical features

Primary tuberculosis. Primary disease, seldom seen in Western Europe and the USA, consists of an initial febrile illness with erythema nodosum and/or phlyctenular conjunctivitis. Within 12 months of the primary infection, complications of the Ghon focus, including pleural effusion, empyema and bronchopneumonia, may develop. This may be followed by regional lymphadenopathy, including lobar collapse, tuberculous bronchopneumonia and pericardial effusion, which can occur within 2 years of the primary infection, and meningitis and osteomyelitis within 3 years. Late complications, which may appear up to 5 years after the primary infection, include renal and skin disease.

Post-primary tuberculosis ('adult type'). Post-primary disease occurs 5 years or more after the primary infection and develops in only 5% of those infected. It is characterized by extensive tissue necrosis, classically involving the upper lobes of the lung. This is the result of tissue-necrotizing hypersensitivity that is quite distinct from the protective immune reactions seen in most affected individuals. Infected tissue in patients with post-primary tuberculosis is extremely sensitive to necrosis induced by TNF-α and is probably the result of priming by cytokines associated with the type 2 T-helper lymphocyte (Th2) cell maturation pathway.

The main features of post-primary pulmonary tuberculosis are:

- fever and sweating
- cough producing mucoid or purulent sputum
- hemoptysis
- chest wall pain
- dyspnea
- weight loss, lassitude, anorexia
- apical crackles, apical bronchial breathing or wheeze
- pleural effusion
- clubbing.

The radiological features are shown in Figure 4.2.

Diagnosis

Pulmonary tuberculosis is diagnosed following the identification of the organism in a suitable specimen. Such specimens include:

- sputum (expectorated or induced)
- laryngeal swabs
- gastric aspirates after overnight fasting
- pleural fluid
- bronchoalveolar lavage
- blood.

Methods of detecting *Mycobacteria* include microscopic examination, culture on solid media, rapid liquid culture and PCR.

The simplest of these is microscopic examination following Ziehl–Neelsen staining (Figure 4.3) or fluorescent staining with auramine (Figure 4.4) or rhodamine B. This provides a rapid diagnosis of infection with Mycobacterium spp.

Culture methods consist of decontamination of the clinical material (to remove oropharyngeal flora – various disinfectants can be used), followed by incubation on Lowenstein's medium. Inoculated media are

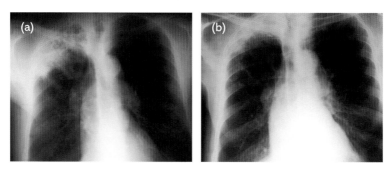

Figure 4.2 (a) Pulmonary tuberculosis in a 47-year-old male immigrant from the Indian subcontinent. In the right upper lobe there is consolidation with cavitation. (b) After three months' therapy with antituberculous chemotherapy. Note the residual fibrosis in the right apex.

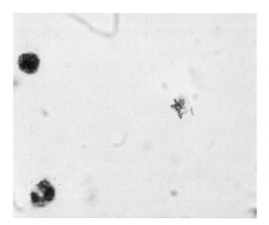

Figure 4.3 Ziehl–Neelsen stain of sputum from the patient in Figure 4.2. The acid-fast bacilli (in the center of the field) are stained pink against a blue background.

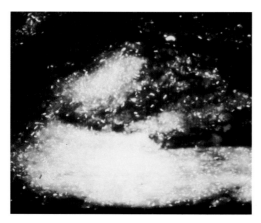

Figure 4.4 Auramine stain of sputum from patient with tuberculosis showing epifluorescence of bacilli. Image courtesy of Dr E Ridgway, Royal Hallamshire Hospital, Sheffield, UK.

incubated for at least 8 weeks and inspected weekly for growth. Most strains of *Mycobacterium tuberculosis* complex produce visible colonies after 4–6 weeks, and are clearly identifiable by their slow growth rate, lack of pigment, temperature sensitivity and sensitivity to *p*-nitrobenzoic acid. Although this technique provides accurate culture diagnosis and sensitivities, it is slow.

Modern techniques to detect growth of *M. tuberculosis* in liquid culture include the BACTEC *Mycobacteria* growth indicator tube (MGIT) system, which can detect organisms in clinical samples in 3–14 days (Figure 4.5). Such systems can provide antibiotic susceptibility data fast. DNA amplification by PCR is also increasingly used and has a sensitivity of 100% in smear-positive sputa. It can rapidly detect antibiotic resistance markers, a particularly useful technique when PCR is used in conjunction with liquid culture.

Serodiagnostic techniques have been disappointing because of lack of specificity.

Tuberculin testing measures an individual's sensitivity to tuberculin protein, and conversion from a negative to a positive tuberculin test indicates recent infection. A number of factors may depress reactivity, including:

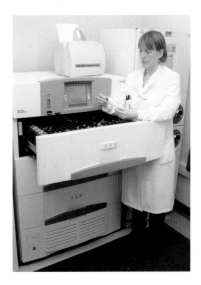

Figure 4.5 Modern methods of culture of *M. tuberculosis* include the BACTEC MGIT system.

- advanced disease
- old age
- malnutrition
- immunosuppression, including that caused by HIV infection
- intrinsic 'poor reactors'
- infectious mononucleosis and other recent viral infections
- recent administration of live viral vaccines
- sarcoidosis
- corticosteroid therapy.

Mantoux test. In the Mantoux test as it is used in the UK, 0.1 mL containing 10 IU of purified protein derivative (PPD), or 1 IU PPD in people likely to react strongly, is injected intracutaneously and the diameter of the resulting induration is measured 48–72 hours later. Reactions more than 10 mm in diameter are positive; those between 5 and 9 mm are doubtful positive. In the USA, the standard dose is 5 IU of intradermal PPD. The lowest cut-off value (5 mm) for the diameter of induration is used for persons with HIV or other immunosuppression, e.g. steroids. For all other persons, the cut-off value is 10 mm, except for those at low risk of TB, in whom it is 15 mm.

Heaf test. In the Heaf test, which is widely used in the UK, a reusable Heaf gun with a disposable head propels six needles into the skin to a depth of 2 mm through a drop of undiluted PPD (100 000 IU/mL). The test is read after 72 hours and graded accordingly (Figure 4.6). A Heaf reaction of at least Grade II is regarded as positive.

Treatment

Experience in the 1950s showed that long periods of therapy with multiple drugs are necessary to avoid relapse caused by the development of resistance. The efficacy of standard chemotherapeutic agents against the functionally different tubercle bacilli is shown in Figure 4.7.

Recommended drug regimens (Table 4.1) consist of an intense 2-month treatment phase in which all but the near-dormant intramacrophage bacilli are killed. This is followed by a 4-month

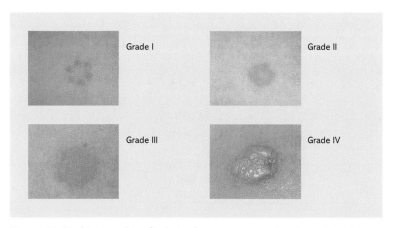

Figure 4.6 Heaf test grading: Grade I – four or more papules at puncture site; Grade II – confluence of the papules into a ring; Grade III – a single large plaque; Grade IV – a plaque with vesicle formation or central necrosis. Reproduced with permission from Dr JA Lunn.

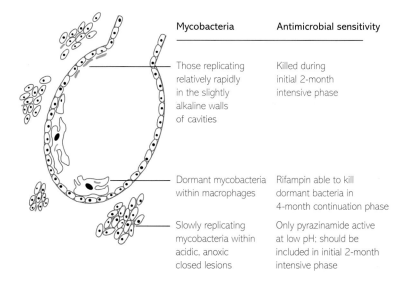

	Mycobacteria	Antimicrobial sensitivity
	Those replicating relatively rapidly in the slightly alkaline walls of cavities	Killed during initial 2-month intensive phase
	Dormant mycobacteria within macrophages	Rifampin able to kill dormant bacteria in 4-month continuation phase
	Slowly replicating mycobacteria within acidic, anoxic closed lesions	Only pyrazinamide active at low pH; should be included in initial 2-month intensive phase

Figure 4.7 A lung infected with *M. tuberculosis* contains at least three functionally distinct mycobacteria with differing sensitivities to antimicrobial agents. Adapted from Grange 1998.

TABLE 4.1

Drug regimens recommended by the WHO for tuberculosis

	Intensive phase (2 months)	Continuation phase (4 months)
Standard regimen – DOTS*	EHRZ daily	HR 3 times/week
	HRZ daily	HR daily
	SHRZ daily	HR daily
	EHRZ daily	HR daily
Intermittent regimens	SHRZ 3 times/week	HRZ 3 times/week
	EHRZ 3 times/week	HRZ 3 times/week

* DOTS, directly observed therapy, short course; E, ethambutol, H, isoniazid, R, rifampin, Z, pyrazinamide, S, streptomycin

continuation phase to eradicate the remaining organisms. The standard regimen recommended by WHO is a short course of directly observed therapy (DOTS). While DOTS ensures compliance, it does require frequent contact between the patient and physician.

The doses and side-effects of commonly used drugs are shown in Table 4.2.

Side-effects. Dangerous hepatotoxicity caused by rifampin (rifampicin in the UK), isoniazid or pyrazinamide can be prevented by regular monitoring of liver function, and interruption of therapy if transaminase levels rise above four times normal. Isoniazid neurotoxicity is avoided by administration of pyridoxine (vitamin B6). Retinopathy associated with ethambutol is possible, but unlikely, at doses of 15 mg/kg or below; it is reversible and can be avoided by regular optometry. Streptomycin (or amikacin) nephrotoxicity and ototoxicity can be avoided by monitoring blood levels and renal function. All patients should be warned about the reduction in efficacy of oral contraceptives during rifampin therapy (due to induction of cytochrome isoenzymes).

Drug-resistant tuberculosis. Factors that point to the possibility of infection with an organism that is resistant to first-line agents include:

- recent immigration from an area with high incidence of MDR tuberculosis (e.g. Pakistan, South-east Asia)
- clinical deterioration despite appropriate therapy
- history of poor compliance.

In the simple case of a patient from a high-risk area with newly diagnosed tuberculosis, the US Advisory Council for the Elimination of Tuberculosis recommends:

- administration of one of the four drug regimens outlined in Table 4.1 under direct supervision
- rapid diagnostic techniques to determine whether the isolate is resistant.

If the organism is proved to be resistant, it may be resistant to a single agent or to two or more agents. Isolated isoniazid-resistant TB should be treated with rifampin, pyrazinamide and ethambutol for 6 months. Isolated rifampin resistance should be treated either with isoniazid and ethambutol for 18 months, *or* isoniazid, pyrazinamide and streptomycin for 9 months. MDR TB (defined as resistant to at least isoniazid and rifampin) should be treated with at least three second-line agents to which the organism is sensitive (Table 4.3). Patients with confirmed MDR tuberculosis should continue treatment for 18–24 months.

Treatment of latent infection

The CDC has recently published guidelines on the management of individuals who are positive on tuberculin skin testing. In the USA, groups targeted for skin testing include:

- HIV-infected persons
- immigrants from countries with high rates of TB
- homeless individuals
- healthcare professionals
- persons living or working in long-term care facilities
- people with conditions that predispose to progression to active disease, e.g. the immunosuppressed, diabetes, chronic renal failure, cancer, silicosis.

Before therapy of a skin-test-positive individual is started, a detailed history should be taken to document any previous treatment of active

65

TABLE 4.2

Doses and adverse effects of drugs commonly used to treat tuberculosis

Drug	Daily dose Adults	Children	Intermittent dose Adults
Isoniazid	300 mg (chemoprophylaxis 5 mg/kg)	10 mg/kg	15 mg/kg (max 750 mg) + pyridoxine, 10 mg daily
Rifampin	< 50 kg: 450 mg > 50 kg: 600 mg	10 mg/kg (max 600 mg)	600–900 mg
Pyrazinamide	< 50 kg: 1.5 g 50–75 kg: 2.0 g > 75 kg: 2.5 g	35 mg/kg	3 times/week: < 50 kg: 2.0 g > 50 kg: 2.5 g Twice/week: < 50 kg: 3.0 g > 50 kg: 3.5 g
Ethambutol	15 mg/kg	If over 12 years of age, as adults	3 times/week: 30 mg/kg Twice/week: 45 mg/kg
Streptomycin	< 50 kg: 0.75 g > 50 kg: 1.0 g, or 0.75 g if over 40 years of age	20 mg/kg	< 50 kg: 0.75 g > 50 kg: 1.0 g
Thiacetazone	150 mg	4 mg/kg	Unsuitable

disease or latent infection, and a chest radiograph should be taken. If a decision is made to treat, the standard regimen is isoniazid 5 mg/kg/day, up to a maximum of 300 mg/day, for 9 months.

Bacille Calmette–Guérin (BCG) vaccine contains a live, attenuated strain of *M. bovis*. Its efficacy varies remarkably from country to country, but in children in the UK, it has a protective efficacy of

Children	Common side-effects	Drug interactions
15 mg/kg (max 750 mg) + pyridoxine, 10 mg daily	Peripheral neuropathy; cutaneous hypersensitivity; hepatitis; elevation of hepatic enzymes	Phenytoin
10 mg/kg (max 600 mg)	Nausea and vomiting; hepatitis; toxic reactions in intermittent therapy; orange bodily secretions	Oral contraceptives; coumarin drugs; corticosteroids; digoxin; oral hypoglycemics; methadone
3 times/week 50 mg/kg Twice/week 75 mg/kg	Hepatitis; arthralgia (hyperuricemia); photosensitivity; nausea; anorexia; vomiting	
If over 12 years of age, as adults	Retinopathy (dose-related)	Potentiation of neuromuscular blocking agents
20 mg/kg (max 750 mg)	Giddiness; ataxia; tinnitus; ototoxicity; nephrotoxicity; avoid pregnancy	
Unsuitable	Nausea and vomiting; cutaneous reaction (often severe); conjunctivitis	

70–80% over at least 15 years; it is not advocated for routine use in the USA.

BCG is administered to:

- in the UK, all individuals who are tuberculin-negative, and have no characteristic BCG scar (a tuberculin test is conducted nationwide at age 12–13 years)
- health professionals

TABLE 4.3

Treatment of drug-resistant tuberculosis: second-line agents

Agent	Dose	Common adverse events
Ethionamide Prothionamide	< 50 kg: 0.75 g in divided doses (to avoid nausea) > 50 kg: 1.0 g in divided doses	Gastrointestinal; metallic taste in mouth
Sodium paraaminosalicylate (PAS)	10–12 g/day in two equal doses	Gastrointestinal; fever; rash
Cycloserine	250 mg twice/day increasing to 250 mg 3 times/day	Confusion; convulsions; suicide
Aminoglycosides (kanamycin, viomycin)	< 50 kg: 0.75 g > 50 kg: 1.0 g, or 0.75 g if over 40 years of age Monitor serum urea, creatinine and electrolyte concentrations	As for streptomycin (Table 4.2), but ototoxicity less common
Capreomycin	As for aminoglycosides	
Ciprofloxacin	250–500 mg twice/day	Relatively well tolerated

- vets
- prison staff
- contacts of patients with active tuberculosis who have two consecutive negative tuberculin tests.

BCG is contraindicated in:

- patients receiving corticosteroids or other immunosuppressive therapy
- HIV-infected individuals
- hematological malignancies
- pregnant women.

BCG vaccination can result in a positive tuberculin skin test, so it is impossible to determine whether a vaccinated person has induration because of recent infection or previous BCG vaccination. However, the CDC recommends that a history of BCG vaccination should be ignored when a tuberculin skin test is administered and interpreted.

Pulmonary tuberculosis – Key points

- New, rapid diagnostic tests are now routine.
- Recent guidelines for the management of TB, MDR TB and latent infection are available.
- TB is common in HIV infection, especially in Africa.

Key references

CDC/ATS Joint Guidelines. Targeted tuberculin testing and treatment of latent tuberculosis infection. *Am J Respir Crit Care Med* 2000;161: S221–47.

Grange JM. Tuberculosis. In: Collier L, Balows A, Sussman M, eds. *Topley & Wilson's Microbiology and Microbial Infections*. Balows A, Duerden B, vol eds. *Vol 2. Systematic Bacteriology*. 9th edn. London: Arnold, 1998:391–418.

Joint Tuberculosis Committee of the British Thoracic Society. Control and prevention of tuberculosis in the United Kingdom: Code of practice 2000. *Thorax* 2000;55:887–901.

Bronchiectasis

Bronchiectasis refers to irreversible abnormal dilation of the bronchi accompanied by suppurative inflammation that is subject to infective exacerbations. Thickened, infected mucus is produced continuously and must be expectorated in order to prevent exacerbations developing. During an infective exacerbation, large quantities of purulent sputum are produced. The most common causes of bronchiectasis are severe parenchymal infections of the lung, including pertussis and measles in childhood and, most importantly in the developing world, tuberculosis (Table 5.1).

Pathogenesis. The initial feature is damage to the conducting airways of the lung and interference with mucociliary clearance. Once bronchiectasis is present, repeated infections serve to maintain a vicious cycle of inflammation and damage to the already compromised airway, which leads to further infection (Figure 5.1). The sputum of patients

TABLE 5.1

Common causes of bronchiectasis

- Childhood infections, including pertussis and measles
- Tuberculosis
- Foreign bodies
- Carcinoma
- Allergic bronchopulmonary aspergillosis (ABPA)
- Rheumatoid disease
- Immunoglobulin deficiency (including subclass deficiency, particularly IgG_2, IgG_4)
- Ciliary abnormalities (e.g. Kartagener's syndrome)
- Cystic fibrosis

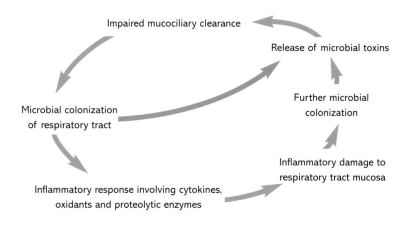

Figure 5.1 Vicious cycle hypothesis of pathogenesis of bronchiectasis. Adapted from Cole PJ, Wilson R. Host-microbial interrelationships in respiratory infection. *Chest* 1989;95:217S–83.

with bronchiectasis is chronically infected with the following pathogens:
- *H. influenzae*
- *S. pneumoniae*
- *S. aureus*
- *P. aeruginosa.*

Extracellular products of each of these organisms are capable of exacerbating the disruption in mucociliary clearance, either by a direct effect on the epithelial cells of the airway, or by induction of an inflammatory infiltrate. In established disease, chronic infection with *P. aeruginosa* is associated with a particularly poor prognosis.

Clinical features. The most prominent clinical feature of bronchiectasis is a cough that produces large quantities (e.g. a cupful per day) of purulent phlegm (which, on standing, shows characteristic sputum layering), together with fatigue and wheeze. During exacerbations, patients may be breathless, wheezy and febrile. In severe cases, clubbing is present.

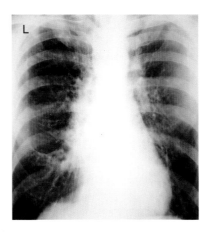

Figure 5.2 A chest radiograph from a patient with Kartagener's syndrome ('L' indicates the left side of the patient's chest). The patient demonstrated situs inversus with dextrocardia. The lung fields show tramlines and ring shadows. Reproduced courtesy of Dr R Peck, Royal Hallamshire Hospital, Sheffield, UK.

Diagnosis is usually clinically obvious in patients with extensive bronchiectasis, but in patients with relatively minor, focal disease, the diagnosis may be suggested by recurrent lower respiratory tract infections that are slow to clear. The diagnosis is essentially radiological. The chest radiograph may be normal, or demonstrate abnormal thick, dilated bronchi producing ring shadows or tramlines (Figure 5.2). High-resolution computed tomography (HRCT) scanning of the thorax may demonstrate dilated airways and bronchial wall thickening (Figure 5.3).

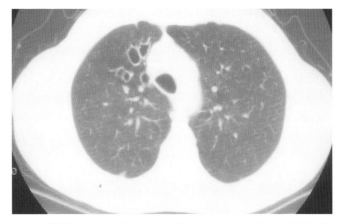

Figure 5.3 HRCT scan showing grossly dilated airways with bronchial-wall thickening in a patient with bronchiectasis. Reproduced with permission from Dr R Nakielny, Royal Hallamshire Hospital, Sheffield, UK.

In patients with newly diagnosed bronchiectasis, a number of investigations may elucidate the cause. These include:

- immunoglobulins, including subclasses (total immunoglobulin can be normal in patients with a subclass deficiency)
- rheumatoid factor
- *Aspergillus* precipitins
- microscopy/EM studies to identify ciliary abnormalities.

The distribution of the bronchiectasis is related to the initiating cause. In general, bronchiectasis resulting from a generalized abnormality, such as a ciliary abnormality, cystic fibrosis or hypogammaglobulinemia, is widespread and affects both the proximal and distal airways. In contrast, bronchiectasis resulting from tuberculosis or impaction of a foreign body is usually localized to a lobe or bronchopulmonary segment; upper lobe involvement is particularly common following allergic bronchopulmonary aspergillosis and tuberculosis.

During exacerbations, sputum should always be sent to the laboratory for microbiological examination to determine antibiotic susceptibilities and, in particular, to identify infection with β-lactamase-secreting *H. influenzae* and also *P. aeruginosa*, both of which are unlikely to respond to aminopenicillins.

Management. The mainstay of treatment of bronchiectasis is drainage, which can be provided by a combination of postural drainage (Figure 5.4) and physiotherapy. These measures reduce the frequency of exacerbations and the need for antibiotic therapy if conducted on a daily basis.

Antibiotic therapy. Beta-lactams do not penetrate bronchiectatic tissue well at conventional doses, but high doses of amoxicillin (e.g. 6 g/day) are more effective in terminating exacerbations. High doses of oral cephalosporins or ciprofloxacin are also effective when β-lactamase-producing strains are isolated. In outpatients colonized with *P. aeruginosa*, intermittent use of high-dose oral ciprofloxacin for exacerbations is the mainstay of therapy.

Long-term oral antibiotics are well tolerated and can lead to symptomatic improvement, but ciprofloxacin-resistant *P. aeruginosa*

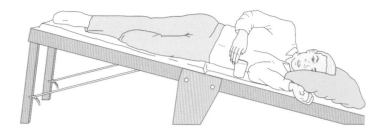

Figure 5.4 Postural drainage in the management of bronchiectasis. The patient is tipped at an angle of approximately 20°.

may be troublesome. The use of a prophylactic aminoglycoside given by nebulizer (e.g. nebulized gentamicin) is of dubious value, but there are numerous anecdotal reports of success.

In extremely severe exacerbations requiring hospitalization, an intravenous antibiotic effective against *H. influenzae* and *P. aeruginosa* (e.g. ceftazidime, aminoglycosides or ciprofloxacin) is indicated.

Surgery. Surgical excision of bronchiectatic tissue was widely used in the past, particularly in patients with localized disease. Nowadays, however, it is seldom performed, because thin-cut CT scanning has shown that most patients have widespread disease to some extent. In patients with extremely severe bronchiectasis that is life-threatening, heart–lung transplantation may be indicated.

Cystic fibrosis

Cystic fibrosis is an autosomal-recessive disease resulting from a mutation of the cystic fibrosis gene on chromosome 7. Approximately 5% of Caucasians carry the mutation; about 6000 people in the UK and 30 000 in the USA are affected. The mutation results in absence or poor functioning of the cystic fibrosis transmembrane regulator (CFTR) protein. This leads to pancreatic dysfunction and an associated abnormality of airway secretions, in which mucins form thick gels with altered rheological properties. The resulting thick, tenacious sputum in the airways causes obstruction that leads to recurrent infection.

Clinical features. Infants present with:
- meconium ileus at birth
- diarrhea or malabsorption in infancy
- failure to thrive
- progressive cough
- recurrent pneumonia.

Pulmonary disease may, in some cases, be relatively mild or even present for the first time in adult life. In most young children with moderately severe disease, acute exacerbations occur, with increased sputum production, cyanosis, dyspnea, fever and weight loss. Patients also suffer from nasal polyposis and chronic sinusitis.

Microbiology. The first pathogen to colonize children with cystic fibrosis is *S. aureus*. Exotoxins of *S. aureus* induce bronchial-wall injury and abscess formation. The intense inflammatory response to *S. aureus* ultimately leads to tissue destruction and bronchiectasis.

The defect in mucociliary clearance in these patients, together with injury due to staphylococcal infections, permits colonization by other bacteria including *P. aeruginosa*. Patients are at first colonized by non-mucoid strains, but later, mucoid variants emerge. These strains cannot be completely eradicated, despite the high antibody levels observed in patients and the intensive antibiotic therapy that they receive. Once *P. aeruginosa* infection is established, it is impossible to eradicate, and proteases produced by the bacteria cause significant damage to the airways. *P. aeruginosa* pigments interfere with mucociliary function. Other products, including the hemolysin rhamnolipid, also reduce mucociliary transport.

Other organisms often isolated from the sputum of cystic fibrosis patients include non-typable *H. influenzae* and *S. pneumoniae*. *Burkholderia cepacia* also colonizes these patients and is transmissible between close contacts. This organism can occasionally be responsible for a fulminating septicemia. It is intrinsically highly resistant to antibiotics including those effective against *P. aeruginosa*, but is usually sensitive to trimethoprim–sulfamethoxazole and chloramphenicol. A range of other bacteria, including the Enterobacteriaceae and *Stenotrephomonas (Xanthomonas) maltophilia*, can also colonize such patients. In patients with severe disease, *Candida albicans*, *Aspergillus* and environmental mycobacteria can also occasionally be isolated in the sputum.

Diagnosis. The diagnosis rests on the clinical presentation, nasal potential difference and sweat chloride concentrations, and can be confirmed by genotyping. A sweat chloride concentration of over 70 mEq/L usually indicates cystic fibrosis. In adults, such investigations may be prompted by recurrent pneumonias or by unexplained isolation of *P. aeruginosa* from an adolescent or an adult with bronchiectasis.

Management. Daily postural drainage and physiotherapy are mandatory in patients with established bronchiectasis due to cystic fibrosis. Once disease is established, some physicians attempt to suppress sputum colonization by long-term administration of antibiotics including:
- oral cephalosporins
- oral chloramphenicol
- trimethoprim–sulfamethoxazole
- amoxicillin–clavulanic acid.

However, such an approach has not been proved to be effective. Most centers treat only acute exacerbations of pulmonary infection, with inclusion of empirical anti-*Pseudomonas* and anti-*S. aureus* antibiotics. Appropriate intravenous therapy might include:
- a β-lactam plus an aminoglycoside
- ceftazidime plus an aminoglycoside
- ciprofloxacin
- an anti-*Pseudomonas* penicillin plus aminoglycoside
- an anti-*Pseudomonas* penicillin with a β-lactamase inhibitor.

In principle, antibiotic regimens should be rotated, and directed by sputum evaluation and microbial sensitivities.

Intravenous therapy administered at home is now widely used in these patients. Appropriate antibiotics include ceftazidime, the penems, monobactams, and β-lactam + β-lactamase inhibitors. Unfortunately, monotherapy can result in the spread of resistant organisms (e.g. *P. aeruginosa*), particularly with the use of ceftazidime, imipenem and aztreonam.

Oral quinolones, such as ciprofloxacin, have permitted more flexible management of exacerbations and are now routinely used in children with cystic fibrosis in most centers. Although resistant *P. aeruginosa* can emerge during therapy with ciprofloxacin, in-vitro susceptibility of isolates returns when the quinolones are withheld for 3 months. Nebulized antibiotics, including tobramycin, have been shown to eradicate *P. aeruginosa*, but emergence of resistant strains during therapy has been a problem.

Other modes of therapy under evaluation include DNAase, which reduces sputum viscosity, and amiloride and triphosphate nucleotides, which restore salt and water secretions.

Bronchiectasis and cystic fibrosis – Key points

- Regular drainage and physiotherapy are critical for reduction in frequency of exacerbations.
- Early aggressive antibiotic therapy of exacerbations is important.
- Cystic fibrosis should be managed in specialized centers.

Key references

Barker AF. Bronchiectasis. *N Engl J Med* 2002;346:1383–93.

Couriel J. Assessment of the child with recurrent chest infections. *Br Med Bull*. 2002;61:115–32.

Pulmonary disease in an immunocompromised host may be due to a number of infectious or non-infectious causes that can each occur with or without fever.

Non-infectious causes

Non-infectious causes of pulmonary infiltrates include:

- pulmonary edema
- cytotoxic drug-induced lung injury (e.g. bleomycin injury)
- pulmonary hemorrhage
- radiation pneumonitis
- pulmonary infiltration of the underlying malignancy
- organizing pneumonitis.

Large-volume infusions of chemotherapeutic agents can lead to pulmonary edema, particularly in severely ill or septic patients with impaired renal function or other factors that increase susceptibility to this condition. Interstitial lung injury induced by cytotoxic drugs is usually most severe after cumulative doses of 150 mg or more, but can occur at lower doses following combination chemotherapy.

Radiation pneumonitis usually occurs at least 1 month after irradiation, in a pattern that exactly traces the therapeutic field. Infiltrative malignancies (e.g. lymphangitic carcinomatosis, non-Hodgkin's lymphoma) are generally insidious, and evidence of malignant spread elsewhere (for instance, to the liver or bone) may be seen.

Infectious causes

In general, susceptibility to infection can be classified according to the underlying defect of innate or specific-acquired immunity. Extracellular pathogens, such as certain bacteria or fungi, are able to flourish in patients with functional defects in complement, antibodies or phagocytes (e.g. neutrophils or macrophages). Defense against intracellular pathogens requires efficient activity of T-helper cells or cytotoxic T-cells. Infections associated with specific common defects of the inflammatory or immunological response are shown in Table 6.1.

TABLE 6.1

Infections associated with common defects in inflammatory or immunological responses

Host defect	Examples of disease associated with defect	Common infections
Neutropenia	• Hematological malignancies • Cytotoxic chemotherapy	• Gram-negative bacillary pneumonia • S. aureus pneumonia • Invasive Aspergillus infection
Ineffective macrophage phagocytosis	• Systemic lupus erythematosus (SLE) • Diabetes • Non-Hodgkin's lymphoma	Pneumonia due to: • S. pneumoniae • H. influenzae • S. aureus
Complement deficiency	• SLE • Congenital deficiency	Pneumonia due to: • S. pneumoniae • Pseudomonas spp.
Antibody deficiency	• Hypogammaglobulinemia • Multiple myeloma • Chronic lymphocytic leukemia	Pneumonia due to: • S. pneumoniae • H. influenzae • S. aureus • Klebsiella spp. • Gram-negative bacilli
T-lymphocyte deficiency/ dysfunction	• Hodgkin's disease • AIDS • Organ transplantation • High-dose corticosteroid therapy	• Pneumocystis carinii • Cytomegalovirus • Herpes simplex virus • Mycobacterium spp. • Aspergillus spp. • Cryptococcus neoformans • Legionella spp. • Nocardia spp.

Clinical features

Patients with an infective pneumonitis usually have fever together with cough and dyspnea.

Time course of illness. Individual infections vary in their severity and speed of evolution. In AIDS, *Pneumocystis carinii* pneumonia (PCP) has an indolent course with symptoms extending over 3–4 weeks. In contrast, PCP in patients with other immunocompromising disorders (e.g. Hodgkin's disease) is acute and fulminant. Similarly, bacterial infections are rapid and aggressive, particularly in the neutropenic host. Some infections evolve over 1–2 weeks; these include cytomegalovirus (CMV), pneumonitis in organ transplant patients, *Aspergillus* infections in neutropenic patients, and cryptococcosis in patients with AIDS. Mycobacterial infections and other chronic bacterial infections (e.g. *Nocardia*) tend to evolve slowly.

Degree of immunosuppression. Pneumonitis in neutropenic patients tends to occur when the absolute neutrophil count is less than 0.5×10^9/liter. In AIDS patients, pneumonitis due to *P. carinii* or *Cryptococcus neoformans* is generally seen when the CD4 count falls below 0.2×10^9/liter, and *Mycobacterium intracellulare* disease when the CD4 count falls below 0.05×10^9/liter.

Time of onset. In organ transplant recipients, CMV pneumonia tends to occur 1–6 months after surgery, and does not occur before or after this period.

Physical examination of the chest may be normal even when the chest radiograph reveals extensive infiltration. A number of features may, however, be helpful in the assessment of etiology and severity of pneumonitis.

- Respiratory rate is a sensitive marker of severity.
- Subtle features (e.g. rales) may become apparent before the chest radiograph becomes abnormal.
- The presence of localized wheeze may indicate a partially obstructed bronchus, suggestive of neoplastic infiltration.

- The presence of a pleural rub in an aggressive pneumonitis suggests bacterial or *Aspergillus* infection, but is seldom present in PCP.

Chest radiographs may reveal characteristic features (Figure 6.1; Table 6.2).

Laboratory diagnosis

In general, samples should be taken for laboratory diagnosis in parallel with the institution of empirical therapy. Sputum and blood culture will yield a diagnosis in a small number of patients. Serology for CMV, cryptococcal antigen or *L. pneumophila* is relatively unhelpful in the acute phase of the illness.

The following lung-sampling or biopsy techniques are the most useful for diagnosis.

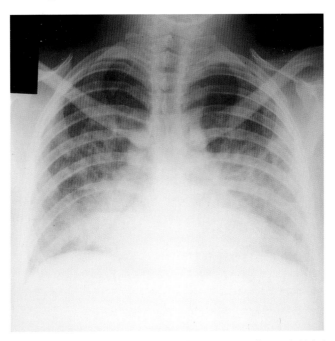

Figure 6.1 This patient presented 6 weeks after renal transplant with high fever and dry cough. Immunofluorescence of bronchoalveolar lavage was positive for cytomegalovirus, and transbronchial biopsy revealed cells with 'owl's-eye' inclusion bodies typical of CMV infection.

TABLE 6.2

Characteristic radiographic features of pulmonary disease in the immunocompromised host

Diffuse infiltrates

- *Pneumocystis carinii* pneumonia (PCP)
- Cytomegalovirus pneumonitis
- Pulmonary edema
- Lymphangitic carcinomatosis

Nodular or cavitating lesions

- Mycobacterial infections
- Cryptococcal infections
- *Nocardia* infections
- Invasive *Aspergillus* infection

Focal infiltrates

- Bacterial pneumonias
- *Cryptococcus neoformans*
- Radiation pneumonitis
- Invasive *Aspergillus* infection

- Induced sputum using 3% nebulized saline can reveal a diagnosis in patients with diffuse infiltrates on the chest radiograph, particularly in patients with AIDS. This technique may reveal infection with *P. carinii* or *Mycobacterium* spp.
- Bronchoalveolar lavage has a sensitivity of greater than 90% in detecting PCP in patients with AIDS and a sensitivity of 40–80% in patients with other immunocompromising illnesses.
- Transbronchial biopsy can be conducted at the same time as bronchoalveolar lavage. It is particularly useful in the diagnosis of diffuse pulmonary infiltrates due to infection.
- Open lung biopsy is the gold standard for diagnosis and provides a diagnosis in more than 90% of patients.

Techniques. Sputum and bronchial washings can be subjected to the following staining techniques:
- Gram stain to identify conventional pathogens
- Ziehl–Neelsen stain to identify *Mycobacterium* spp. and *Nocardia*
- india ink to identify *Cryptococcus*
- potassium hydroxide to identify *Aspergillus* and *Mucor*
- methenamine silver stain to identify *P. carinii*
- Wright–Giemsa stain to identify CMV
- monoclonal antibodies (direct immunofluorescence) to identify *Legionella*, *P. carinii*, CMV and herpes simplex virus (HSV)
- PCR to detect CMV and HSV.

Culture techniques include:
- blood/lysed blood agar to identify conventional pathogens
- Lowenstein–Jensen medium to identify *Mycobacterium* spp.
- Sabouraud agar to identify *Mucor*, *Candida*, *Nocardia* and *Cryptococcus*
- cell culture to identify CMV and herpes simplex virus.

Management

Unfortunately, the low yield of non-invasive investigations and the frailty of patients often necessitates a full empirical approach. An organized strategy has been suggested by Fanta and Pennington (Figure 6.2).

In patients with focal infiltrates, particularly neutropenic patients, antibiotic cover against Gram-negative bacilli (including *P. aeruginosa*) and *Staphylococci* is necessary. Suitable combinations include:
- a third-generation cephalosporin (e.g. ceftazidime) plus an aminoglycoside
- a broad-spectrum penicillin (e.g. ticarcillin or piperacillin) plus an aminoglycoside plus a glycopeptide (e.g. vancomycin)
- piperacillin/tazobactam plus ciprofloxacin.

In patients who have bilateral pulmonary infiltrates, particularly those with a type of immunosuppression that generally favors overgrowth with *P. carinii*, empirical therapy with trimethoprim–sulfamethoxazole is warranted, together with therapy directed against *L. pneumophila*, which commonly presents with bilateral infiltrates.

83

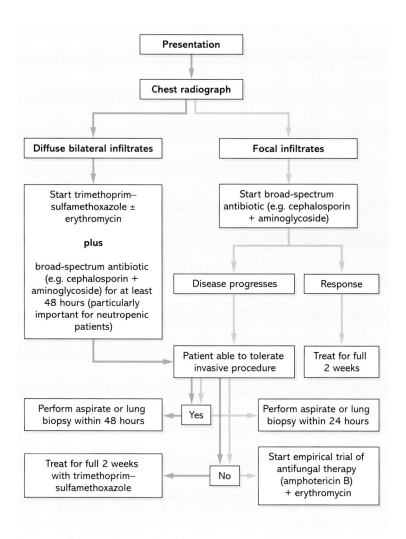

Figure 6.2 Suggested approach to the management of fever and pulmonary infiltrates in the immunocompromised host. Adapted with permission from Fanta CH, Pennington JE in Pennington 1994.

Every effort should be made to make a diagnosis by induction of sputum, bronchoalveolar lavage or lung biopsy in order to spare the patient 2 weeks of unnecessary therapy; in some centers, however, it is common practice to wait and see whether there is a response to empirical therapy before employing invasive diagnostic techniques.

The clinical condition of some patients with localized infiltrates is too severe to warrant invasive diagnostic techniques. If these patients fail to respond to initial empirical antimicrobial therapy, an alternative choice is to initiate erythromycin together with empirical antifungal therapy (amphotericin B).

Pneumonia in the immunocompromised host – Key points

- The microbiological diagnosis is sometimes suggested by the immune defect of the host.
- An extended number of microbiological tests should be performed on respiratory samples.
- Empiric therapy should be commenced immediately without waiting for positive microbiological tests.

Key references

Pennington JE, ed. *Respiratory Infections. Diagnosis and Management*. 3rd edn. New York: Raven, 1994.

The lung is an important site of disease in patients with HIV infection. Pulmonary complications can occur at any stage of the illness (Figure 7.1; Table 7.1).

In developed countries, the most common problems involving the lung are acute bronchitis, pneumococcal pneumonia and PCP. In general, pulmonary complications are related to the immune status (CD4 count) and the risk factor associated with HIV infection for each individual. In the USA, the Pulmonary Complications of HIV Infection Study has shown that most individuals with early HIV disease experience relatively minor respiratory problems, including upper respiratory tract infections (e.g. sinusitis and acute bronchitis). Those

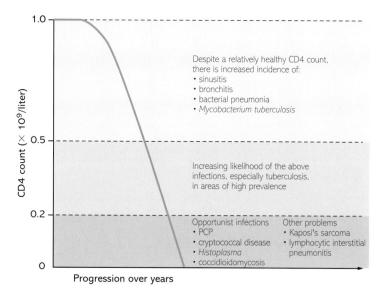

PCP = *Pneumocystis carinii* pneumonia

Figure 7.1 Relationship between the natural history of HIV infection and pulmonary complications.

TABLE 7.1
Pulmonary complications in HIV infection

Bacteria	Fungal infection
Mycobacterium tuberculosis	Pneumocystis carinii
Mycobacterium kansasii	Cryptococcus neoformans
Mycobacterium avium complex	Histoplasma capsulatum
Streptococcus pneumoniae	Coccidioides immitis
Haemophilus influenzae	Aspergillus fumigatus
Staphylococcus aureus	Penicillium marneffei
Moraxella catarrhalis	
Pseudomonas aeruginosa	**Viruses**
Nocardia asteroides	Cytomegalovirus
Rhodococcus equi	Herpes simplex virus
	Lymphocytic interstitial
Lung tumors	**pneumonitis**
Kaposi's sarcoma	
Non-Hodgkin's lymphoma	

with CD4 counts between 0.2×10^9/liter and 0.5×10^9/liter are at increased risk of developing PCP and bacterial pneumonia, especially due to *S. pneumoniae*. In severely immunocompromised patients (CD4 $< 0.2 \times 10^9$/liter), PCP and bacterial pneumonia occur at much higher rates, even when chemoprophylaxis (e.g. trimethoprim–sulfamethoxazole) is used.

Changes in pulmonary manifestation of HIV infection in the era of highly active antiretroviral therapy (HAART). Even before the use of highly active antiretroviral therapy, there were downward trends in certain pulmonary manifestations of HIV infection, especially PCP (see Figure 7.2), largely because of greatly improved diagnostic techniques, physicians' improved awareness, and improved expertise with prophylaxis and therapy such as trimethoprim–sulfamethoxazole.

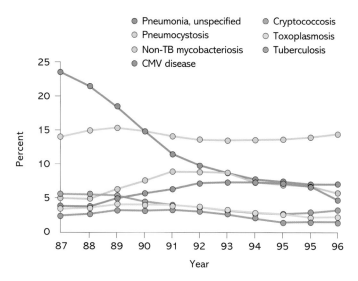

Figure 7.2 Trends in the percentage of deaths with selected infectious diseases among persons dying of HIV infection, 1987–1997. Source: Centers for Disease Control and Prevention, USA.

Since HAART became routine, there have been further notable trends in pulmonary manifestations. *Pneumocystis carinii* pneumonia has become relatively less common, whilst bacterial pneumonia and non-Hodgkin's lymphoma have become relatively more common. However, new HIV infections continue to occur, and physicians must remain vigilant for the occurrence of PCP in newly presenting patients.

Diagnosis

The CD4 count is an important guide in the evaluation of patients with pulmonary symptoms and signs. However, the clinical history together

Figure 7.3 (facing page) Diagnostic algorithm for evaluation of respiratory symptoms in an HIV-infected patient at risk for *P. carinii* pneumonia and bacterial pneumonia. HIV, human immunodeficiency virus; HRCT, high-resolution computed tomograph; GGO, ground-glass opacities; DLCO, diffusing capacity for carbon monoxide; Rx, treatment, AFB, acid-fast bacilli; BAL, bronchoalveolar lavage; KS, Kaposi's sarcoma; CT, computed tomography; FNA, fine-needle aspirate. From Huang L et al., 2000.

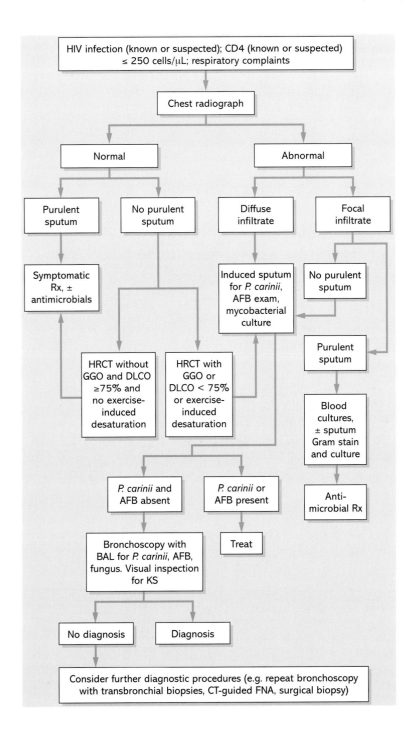

with a few simple investigations can usually establish the diagnosis (Figure 7.3). The relevant clinical features that may help to distinguish the more common pulmonary complications are listed in Table 7.2.

Investigations. An initial chest radiograph may provide important diagnostic clues (Table 7.3; Figures 7.4 and 7.5). In patients with normal chest radiographs, indicators of significant pulmonary disease include:

TABLE 7.2

Characteristic clinical features of common pulmonary complications

Pneumocystis carinii pneumonia

- Absence of prophylaxis
- Insidious onset
- Prodrome of fevers, night sweats, weight loss and oral candidiasis
- Dry cough
- Retrosternal irritation on deep breath
- Absence of pleuritic chest pain
- CD4 count $< 0.2 \times 10^9$/liter
- Reduced carbon monoxide diffusion capacity

Bacterial pneumonia

- Severe and abrupt onset
- Productive cough
- Pleuritic chest pain
- High peripheral white blood cell count

Tuberculosis

Early disease

- Cough with or without hemoptysis
- Weight loss
- Localized or diffuse lung abnormalities on the chest radiograph

Late disease

- Pronounced constitutional symptoms
- Diffuse infiltrates on the chest radiograph

Kaposi's sarcoma

- Insidious onset of dyspnea
- Persistent cough
- Presence of lesions elsewhere

Fungal diseases (*Histoplasma*, *Coccidioides*)

- Residence in endemic area

TABLE 7.3

Characteristic findings on the chest radiograph in common pulmonary complications of HIV infection

Characteristic finding	Possible diagnosis
Normal	• *Pneumocystis carinii* pneumonia • Disseminated fungal infection
Focal infiltrate	• Bacterial pneumonia • *Mycobacterium tuberculosis* • Fungal pneumonia • *Pneumocystis carinii* pneumonia
Pleural effusion	• Kaposi's sarcoma • Bacterial pneumonia • *Mycobacterium tuberculosis*
Hilar lymphadenopathy	• *Mycobacterium tuberculosis* • Lymphoma
Interstitial infiltrate	• *Pneumocystis carinii* pneumonia • *Mycobacterium tuberculosis* • Lymphocytic interstitial pneumonitis • Bacterial pneumonia

- a carbon monoxide diffusing capacity (DLCO) less than 75% of predicted value
- HRCT scan showing 'ground-glass' opacities
- a greater than 5% drop in oxygen saturation on exercise oximetry.

Respiratory secretions can be obtained either by induction of sputum production using ultrasonic nebulization of 3% saline, or by bronchoalveolar lavage. The secretions should be examined by:

- microbiological staining for *P. carinii* (e.g. modified Giemsa, methenamine silver, toluidine blue O)
- Ziehl–Neelsen or auramine staining for *Mycobacterium* spp.
- culture for mycobacteria, other bacteria, fungi and viruses
- monoclonal antibody-based immunofluorescence assays for *P. carinii*, herpes simplex virus, CMV and *L. pneumophila*.

Although sputum induction is a valuable investigation, its negative predictive value is relatively poor; thus, patients with a negative induced sputum result should undergo fiber-optic bronchoscopy.

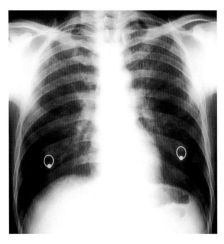

Figure 7.4 This patient presented with a 4-week history of night sweats and dry cough. The chest radiograph shows diffuse bilateral infiltrates. Induced sputum was positive for *P. carinii*, and the patient tested positive for HIV antibody. Reproduced courtesy of Dr R Peck, Royal Hallamshire Hospital, Sheffield, UK.

TABLE 7.4

Treatment of *Pneumocystis carinii* pneumonia

Disease status	Recommended therapy
Mild disease (patient ambulant, $PaO_2 > 8$ kPa)	Trimethoprim, 20 mg/kg/day + sulfamethoxazole, oral, 100 mg/kg every 12 hours for 21 days
Moderate–severe disease ($PaO_2 < 8$ kPa)	Trimethoprim, 20 mg/kg/day, + sulfamethoxazole, i.v., 100 mg/kg/day + prednisone, oral, 40 mg every 12 hours or hydrocortisone, 200 mg, i.v., every 6 hours for 5 days, gradually reducing dose over 21 days

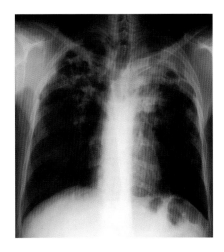

Figure 7.5 This HIV-positive patient presented with 1 month of productive cough and weight loss. The chest radiograph revealed extensive nodular and cavitating consolidation of both upper lobes. Auramine stain of sputum revealed acid-fast bacilli, and culture revealed MDR *M. tuberculosis*.

Alternative therapy	Comments
Dapsone, oral, 100 mg daily, plus trimethoprim, oral, 5 mg/kg every 8 hours	If rash due to trimethoprim–sulfamethoxazole occurs, dose can be reduced to trimethoprim, 15 mg/kg/day, + sulfamethoxazole, 75 mg/kg/day
Atovaquone, oral, 750 mg every 8 hours	
Clindamycin, 450 mg every 6 hours, plus primaquine, oral, 15 mg daily	Clindamycin plus primaquine is highly effective, but often causes severe rash and diarrhea
Pentamidine, i.v., 4 mg/kg every 24 hours	Pentamidine is toxic (rashes, hypoglycemia, renal dysfunction), but is the most potent alternative to trimethoprim–sulfamethoxazole
Clindamycin, i.v., 600 mg every 6 hours, plus primaquine, oral, 15–30 mg daily	
Trimetrexate, i.v., 45 mg/m^2 every 24 hours, plus leucovorin, i.v., 20 mg/m^2 every 6 hours	Trimetrexate is well tolerated, but not as effective as trimethoprim–sulfamethoxazole

TABLE 7.5

Prophylaxis for HIV-related opportunistic infections

Pathogen	Indication for prophylaxis	First choice
Pneumocystis carinii	CD4 count < 0.2 × 10^9/liter Persistent unexplained fever Chronic oropharyngeal candidiasis	Trimethoprim (80–160 mg) –sulfamethoxazole (400–800 mg), oral, daily Dapsone, 100 mg, daily
Mycobacterium tuberculosis	Tuberculin test positive (> 5 mm)	Isoniazid, 300 mg, daily for 12 months
Pneumococcus	All patients	Pneumovax
Haemophilus influenzae	No consensus	Hib vaccine
Influenza	All patients	Influenza vaccine

The combination of bronchoalveolar lavage and transbronchial biopsy will yield a diagnosis in more than 95% of lower respiratory tract infections in patients with AIDS.

Treatment of *Pneumocystis carinii* pneumonia

A number of therapeutic options are available depending on the severity of the disease (Table 7.4); the adjunctive use of corticosteroids in patients with moderate-to-severe *P. carinii* infection is now well established. PCP should be treated for 21 days.

Prevention of pulmonary complications

Pneumocystis carinii infection. All patients with a CD4 count below 0.2×10^9/liter should be offered prophylaxis against *P. carinii*. A major problem is intolerance of some regimens, particularly those involving trimethoprim–sulfamethoxazole. However, a wide range of drugs is available and a suitable regimen can usually be tailored for each patient

Alternatives	Comments
Aerosolized pentamidine Dapsone, 100 mg + pyrimethamine, 25 mg, once weekly	Aerosolized pentamidine should be delivered by Respirgard II® or Fisoneb® nebulizer Trimethoprim–sulfamethoxazole can probably be given 2 or 3 days weekly with high efficacy; single-strength tablets are also effective
	In patients exposed to resistant strains, two-drug regimens using combinations of rifampin, pyrazinamide or a quinolone can be considered
	Trimethoprim–sulfamethoxazole appears to prevent some disease
	Trimethoprim–sulfamethoxazole appears to prevent some disease

(Table 7.5). Nevertheless, trimethoprim–sulfamethoxazole has been the most successful therapy, and breakthrough infections are more commonly seen with aerosolized pentamidine or dapsone.

HIV infection and pulmonary disease – Key points

- Conventional bacterial pneumonias are relatively more common and PCP is relatively less common than before HAART.
- New PCP infections continue to present to physicians.
- Diagnostic algorithms are available for investigation of HIV-infected individuals with pulmonary disease.

Streptococcus pneumoniae. Use of the 23-valent polysaccharide vaccine has been evaluated in patients with HIV. Clinical efficacy is impaired in patients with advanced disease, but the vaccine is routinely offered to new patients, particularly those with early disease.

Mycobacterium tuberculosis. Tuberculin testing should be offered to all patients with HIV infection, but BCG vaccination is absolutely contraindicated. In patients who convert their tuberculin skin test, prophylaxis with isoniazid, 300 mg/day, should be offered.

Key references

Huang L, Hopewell PC. Pulmonary manifestations of HIV infection. In: Wachter RM, Goldman L, Hollander H, eds. *Hospital Medicine*. Philadelphia: Lippincott, Williams & Wilkins, 2000:561–9.

Wolff AJ, O'Donnell EA. Pulmonary manifestations of HIV in the era of highly active antiretroviral therapy. *Chest* 2001;120:1888–93.

Influenza

Pneumonia due to influenza virus infection is most commonly seen in adults. Winter epidemics of influenza A and influenza B occur worldwide. Currently, the H1N1 and H3N2 subtypes are responsible for most epidemics of influenza A, though in the second half of 1997, an outbreak of an avian subtype H5N1 was reported in Hong Kong.

Clinical features. Lower respiratory tract symptoms of pneumonia typically follow 24 hours after the typical 'flu' symptoms with high fever, increasing dyspnea and wheezing. Hemoptysis may be present. The chest radiograph usually shows a diffuse non-lobar infiltrate. Bacterial superinfection of viral pneumonia may occur either simultaneously with the viral pneumonitis or a few days following the initial illness. The bacteria most commonly implicated in such superinfections are *S. pneumoniae*, *S. aureus* and *H. influenzae*.

Diagnosis. The gold standard for diagnosis is culture of virus from respiratory secretions, which are most efficiently obtained by nasopharyngeal aspiration (Figure 8.1). Culture on MDCK or Vero cells generally takes 7–14 days. Rapid diagnostic techniques, such as rapid culture, direct immunofluorescence (which has reduced sensitivity) and PCR tests are currently being adopted as routine laboratory tests.

Antiviral drugs for treatment of influenza. A number of drugs are available for both treatment and prevention of influenza, and these are summarized in Table 8.1.

Amantadine and rimantadine, the older agents, both work by blocking the ion-channel function of the virus protein M2. They are active against influenza A but not against influenza B. Both compounds are effective for treatment of influenza A if treatment is begun within 48 hours of onset, and shorten the illness by approximately one day.

TABLE 8.1

Antiviral agents for influenza

Agent	Trade name	Influenza spectrum
Amantadine	Symmetrel	Type A
Rimantadine*	Flumadine	Type A
Zanamivir	Relenza	Types A and B
Oseltamivir	Tamiflu	Types A and B

* Not available in the UK

They are both given orally, but can cause nausea and vomiting in a small percentage of individuals. Unfortunately, amantadine is associated with a number of unpleasant central nervous system side-effects such as anxiety, depression, insomnia and even hallucinations. Antiviral resistance can develop rapidly during use of either drug, and resistant virus can then be transmitted from the index case to others. Because of their difficult side-effect profile, these drugs have not been deployed for the treatment of community-acquired influenza, but they have been used extensively in chemoprophylaxis.

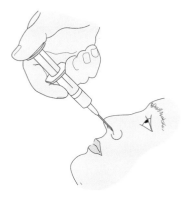

Figure 8.1 Nasopharyngeal wash.

Route of administration	Daily dosage for adults		Most common side-effects
	Prevention	Treatment	
Oral	200 mg	200 mg	Gastrointestinal and central nervous system
Oral	200 mg	200 mg	Gastrointestinal
Oral inhalation	10 mg	20 mg	None
Oral	75 mg	150 mg	Gastrointestinal

Neuraminidase inhibitors. Neuraminidase is essential for the release of newly synthesized virions from infected cells, and inhibition of this enzyme by neuraminidase inhibitors interrupts propagation of influenza virus within the human respiratory tract. Zanamivir is a modification of Neu5Ac2en, a dehydrated neuraminic acid derivative. Oseltamivir is a similar molecule except it has a cyclohexene ring, and a polyglycerol has been replaced with lipophilic side-chains. Zanamivir can only be administered by inhalation, whereas oseltamivir can be taken by mouth. Both of these drugs are active against both influenza virus A and influenza virus B. In clinical trials of treatment of patients with community influenza with oseltamivir or zanamivir, both have been shown to shorten the duration of symptoms by approximately one day. The time gained in returning to normal activities is half a day for laboratory-confirmed cases of influenza. The beneficial effect appears to be confined to patients in whom there is fever, and patients who are treated within 30 hours of symptom onset. Zanamivir has been shown to reduce the frequency of antibiotic prescriptions for lower respiratory tract complications by 40%, but has not reduced prescriptions for presumed upper respiratory tract complications such as sinusitis and otitis. So far, the neuraminidase inhibitors have not been extensively investigated in patients who are at the highest risk of serious complications of influenza, namely the elderly and those with serious cardiopulmonary illness, for example COPD. Although oseltamivir can be given orally, zanamivir must be given via an inhaler device and it is possible that older and very young patients may not be able to deliver the drug effectively. Both drugs appear relatively safe. Zanamivir has very few side-effects, but oseltamivir does cause a significant incidence of nausea.

When used for the treatment of children, inhaled zanamivir has significantly reduced time to alleviation of illness (by approximately one day) and speeded up the return to usual activities. Nebulized zanamivir is available for younger children and infants. A liquid formulation of oseltamivir is effective in children aged 1–10 years and reduces the frequency of complications leading to antibiotic prescriptions.

Antiviral drugs for prophylaxis of influenza. Amantadine and rimantadine have been used for emergency chemoprophylaxis (e.g. in nursing homes or amongst hospital staff in epidemic situations) for many years but are limited by the restriction of their antiviral activity to influenza type A infections. Compared with placebo, neuraminidase inhibitors are approximately 75% effective in the prevention of naturally occurring cases of clinically defined influenza and 60% effective in the prevention of cases of laboratory-confirmed influenza in households in which new cases have been proven by laboratory methods.

Vaccination for prophylaxis of influenza. The influenza vaccine consists of purified hemagglutinin and neuraminidase surface antigens from two circulating Type A influenza viruses and one Type B virus. The Type A virus subunits are changed annually to take account of antigenic drift and are chosen by the World Health Organization. The groups targeted for vaccination include:
- All persons > 65 years of age
- Patients with chronic lung, heart or kidney disease
- People with diabetes mellitus
- Immunosuppressed individuals
- People in long-term residential care facilities.

Respiratory syncytial virus

Respiratory syncytial virus (RSV) is the most common cause of viral pneumonia in children aged 6 months to 3 years in the UK and the USA. It is highly infectious, and spreads rapidly within hospitals and childcare facilities.

Clinical features. Infection can result in bronchiolitis and pneumonia, with prominent wheezing on auscultation and pulmonary infiltrates on the chest radiograph. The disease can be severe in children receiving cytotoxic chemotherapy for malignant disease; however, corticosteroids appear to have no effect on disease severity.

Diagnosis. The diagnosis can be made rapidly by immunofluorescence of nasopharyngeal aspirates (Figure 8.2) or else by culture, which generally takes between 7 and 10 days.

Treatment and prevention. Aerosolized ribavirin is used routinely to treat severe RSV pneumonia in infants and children. In infants treated with ribavirin, blood gases normalize faster and viral shedding decreases. Hyperimmune RSV immunoglobulin is available in the USA for prophylaxis in high-risk infants.

Adenovirus

In most cases, adenovirus pneumonia is caused by serotypes 4, 7 or 21. It occurs in both children and adults.

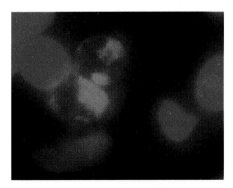

Figure 8.2 Immunofluorescence of nasopharyngeal aspirate from a patient with RSV infection.

Clinical features. Although adenovirus is a common cause of conjunctivitis, this is usually absent in patients with pneumonia. Rather there is gradual onset of illness consisting of fever, dry cough and dyspnea. Occasionally, pleural effusions and rhabdomyolysis are seen in children, but the mortality is very low. Bronchiectasis is a well-documented sequel of childhood adenovirus pneumonia.

Diagnosis is usually either by culture of respiratory secretions or serology. Some centers offer direct immunofluorescence of respiratory secretions.

Treatment. No specific therapy for adenovirus pneumonia has been developed.

Measles

Although respiratory symptoms are fairly common in measles, pneumonia with the appearance of pulmonary infiltrates on the chest radiograph is thought to occur in less than 5% of cases in the developed world; it is much more common in developing countries, where it has been linked to vitamin A deficiency. In most cases, a fine reticular nodular infiltrate can be seen on the chest radiograph. Measles pneumonia can be severe, particularly in malnourished children, in immunocompromised patients and in pregnant women.

Diagnosis can be made by detection of salivary IgM, or by culture of virus from saliva.

Prevention. The incidence of measles and the associated pneumonia has been dramatically reduced in the UK by the use of the live attenuated measles vaccine, which is usually given as part of the MMR (measles, mumps and rubella) vaccination shortly after the first birthday and before school entry.

Treatment is generally supportive or aimed at control of bacterial superinfection.

Varicella zoster virus pneumonia

Chickenpox can be complicated by pneumonia in approximately 10–20% of cases in adults, but is rare in children. It is more common in adults who smoke. Pneumonia usually occurs in those patients with the most severe skin rash and can be severe, particularly in immunocompromised patients and in pregnant women.

Clinical features. Patients with varicella zoster virus (VZV) pneumonia may have a dry cough and dyspnea, and crackles can often be heard on auscultation. The chest radiograph shows a fine nodular infiltrate (Figure 8.3), which calcifies over many years to leave punctate diffuse pulmonary calcification scattered widely throughout the lung fields.

Diagnosis. Chest radiographs should be routinely taken for patients with chickenpox and respiratory signs or symptoms, and digital pulse oximetry should be performed.

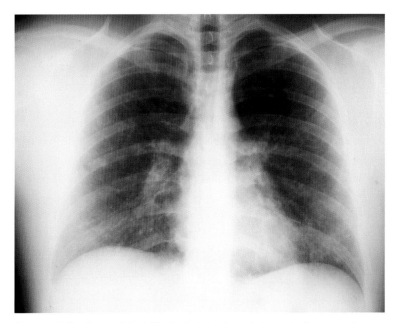

Figure 8.3 The fine nodular infiltrate that develops during varicella zoster virus pneumonia. This calcifies over many years to leave punctate diffuse pulmonary calcification scattered widely throughout the lung fields.

Prevention. A live attenuated VZV vaccine has been developed and is currently being evaluated in the developed world.

Treatment. Aciclovir, 5–10 mg/kg i.v. three times a day, should be administered to patients with VZV pneumonitis. The drug is well tolerated and can be used in pregnancy. Clear benefit has been shown only when the drug has been administered within 48 hours of the onset of the rash.

Cytomegalovirus

CMV pneumonitis is nearly always seen in immunocompromised patients, particularly those who are immunocompromised as part of bone-marrow or renal transplant procedures. CMV pneumonitis may be seen in late-stage AIDS, usually in the context of coexistent *P. carinii* infection.

Clinical features. CMV pneumonitis usually occurs as part of a systemic syndrome, with hepatitis or involvement of the gastrointestinal tract. Patients complain of fever and other systemic symptoms, together with dry cough and dyspnea. The chest radiograph reveals a diffuse interstitial pneumonitis. The illness can be extremely severe and fatal.

Diagnosis is most easily made in patients who have previously been seronegative for CMV and who become seropositive during their acute illness. Culture of the virus from respiratory secretions or the demonstration of the virus by direct immunofluorescence may also aid diagnosis. Lung biopsy may reveal focal areas of inflammatory infiltration including cytomegaly, with 'owl's-eye' inclusions.

Treatment. Ganciclovir, particularly in combination with intravenous immunoglobulin, has improved the prognosis in patients with CMV pneumonitis.

Hantavirus

Hantavirus infection emerged during the 1990s as a cause of severe respiratory illness. The illness has been described in the southwestern

USA, particularly among American Indians. Hantavirus infection probably results from contact with the deer-mouse, but other rodents may also be involved.

Clinical features comprise sudden onset of fever and headache, and some systemic symptoms, together with a rapidly progressing respiratory illness usually beginning with dry cough. The chest radiograph reveals features consistent with adult respiratory distress syndrome. The disease has a high mortality, possibly as great as 50%.

Diagnosis. Antibodies to hantavirus can be detected by ELISA.

Prevention. Rodent control programs should be initiated in areas with outbreaks of hantavirus infection.

Treatment. Intravenous ribavirin has been used successfully in patients with severe hantavirus pneumonitis.

Viral pneumonias – Key points

- Influenza vaccine should be given annually to people in specified risk groups.
- Neuraminidase inhibitors have proven efficacy in treatment and prevention of influenza.
- Serious disease due to RSV in babies can be treated with ribavirin.

Key references

Cox NJ, Subbarao K. Influenza. *Lancet* 1999;354:1277–82.

Palese P, Garcia-Sastre A. Influenza vaccines: present and future. *J Clin Invest* 2002;110:9–13.

Salgado CD, Farr BM, Hall KK, Hayden FG. Influenza in the acute hospital setting. *Lancet Infect Dis* 2002;2:145–55.

The attack on the World Trade Center in New York City on 11 September 2001 changed the Western world and sharply increased concerns about bioterrorism, concerns which had already been growing over the past decade. Areas in which preparations are now under way for dealing with biological weapons include:

- awareness and education
- laboratory diagnosis
- therapeutic interventions
- hospital and community response
- scientific research.

Biological weapons are invisible, odorless and tasteless; and, if properly prepared and disseminated, a small inoculum could infect thousands of persons. It is critically important that medical practitioners recognize the effects of bioweapons so that appropriate prophylactic strategies for patients and for society can be instituted when necessary. Several reviews are listed in the Key references section of this chapter, and websites giving information are listed with other useful addresses at the end of this book.

In the case of a suspected bioterrorist attack, public health officials must be notified as soon as possible during the management of a case.

In 2000, Bartlett and co-workers published Guidelines for the Prevention of Community-Acquired Pneumonia, which included a section on bioterrorism agents that cause pneumonia. Selected bacterial agents included pulmonary anthrax, plague and tularemia. Many of these pathogens are old, but take on a new threat when used as biological weapons. Key features of several agents causing pneumonia are summarized in Table 9.1 and discussed in more detail below.

Bacillus anthracis (anthrax)

Several cases of cutaneous and pulmonary disease due to bioterrorism caused by *B. anthracis* were diagnosed in the United States in the fall of

2001. The source was probably the generation of aerosols from letters containing anthrax spores.

Anthrax is a Gram-positive, spore-forming bacillus that produces disease in cattle, sheep and goats (a heat-cured vaccine produced in 1880 was effective in protecting cattle, but these data are difficult to extrapolate to humans). Three toxins are produced by *B. anthracis*:

- protective antigen
- edema toxin, which inhibits phagocytosis
- lethal toxin, which kills macrophages.

Most of the cases in the United States have been cutaneous. Inhalational disease occurred more commonly in the early 20th century in people handling infected hides, when it was known as 'woolsorter's disease'. In 2001 the disease was often referred to as 'mailsorter's disease'. Inhalational anthrax as a biological weapon is a major concern because of the environmental stability of its spores and the small inoculum needed to cause fulminant infection. In the 1970s the World Health Organization estimated that aerosolization of 60 kg of anthrax from a plane upwind of a large metropolitan city would kill 500 000 people and incapacitate 220 000.

The onset is usually within several days, but may be as long as 6 weeks. Initial symptoms are non-specific and include fever, malaise, chest pain and a non-productive cough which may progress to severe respiratory distress, shock and death. Chest radiography (Figure 9.1) reveals a widened mediastinum with or without pulmonary infiltrates.

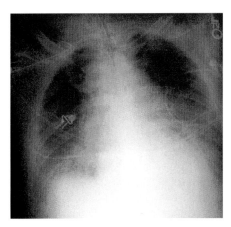

Figure 9.1 Anteroposterior chest radiograph showing the widened mediastinum characteristic of anthrax. A chest radiograph obtained approximately one year before the fatal illness showed a normal mediastinal shadow. Taken with permission from Bush et al. 2001.

TABLE 9.1

Biological warfare agents that would cause pulmonary disease

Feature	Anthrax
Putative agent	*Bacillus anthracis*
Estimated casualties from 50 kg of aerosol over metropolitan area with 5 million persons	250 000 (100 000 would die without treatment)
Mean incubation period	2–6 days (1–42 days)
Clinical findings	Fever, malaise, cough, followed by ARDS and shock
Laboratory findings	Radiographic evidence of widened mediastinum; leukocytosis
Diagnosis	(1) Gram stain of unspun peripheral blood; (2) positive blood culture, negative sputum culture
Treatment	Ciprofloxacin (alternatives: other fluoroquinolones,* doxycycline or penicillin, if susceptible)
Duration of therapy	60 days
Isolation	Standard (no person-to-person spread)
Mortality	> 95% without therapy; 80% with therapy
Prophylaxis after exposure	Ciprofloxacin, amoxicillin or doxycycline
Duration of prophylaxis	60 days
Vaccine	Likely to be effective in postexposure setting, but no vaccine is currently available for civilian use
Person-to-person transmission	None

DIC, diffuse intravascular coagulation; CSF, cerebrospinal fluid
* Ciprofloxacin, levofloxacin, ofloxacin, grepafloxacin or sparfloxacin
Taken with permission from Bartlett JG et al. 2000

Plague	Tularemia
Yersinia pestis	*Francisella tularensis*
150 000 (36 000 would die without treatment)	250 000 (17 000 would die without treatment)
2–5 days (1–6 days)	3–5 days (1–21 days)
Fever, malaise, cough ± bloody sputum, followed by shock	Fever, prostration, cough
Radiographic evidence of patchy or consolidated infiltrate; leukocytosis; DIC	Radiographic evidence of focal pneumonia + hilar nodes
Gram-negative bipolar coccobacillus on stain and culture of blood, sputum, CSF	Culture of blood, sputum, and pharyngeal specimen (high risk to laboratory personnel; use BL-3 facility in suspected cases)
Streptomycin or gentamicin (alternatives: tetracyclines or fluoroquinolones*)	Doxycycline, streptomycin or gentamicin; chloramphenicol
10 days	14 days
Respiratory precautions until treated for 48 h	Standard (person-to-person spread is rare)
~100% unless treated in < 24h	35% without treatment; 1%–2% with treatment
Doxycycline or fluoroquinolone*	Doxycycline
7 days	14 days
Not effective for plague pneumonia	Live vaccine is investigational new drug under study
Patient can be contagious to close contacts until treated for 48 h	None

Blood cultures may be positive, and smears of peripheral blood white-cell buffy coats may demonstrate Gram-positive bacilli (Figure 9.2). Mortality rates are often > 50% with treatment and > 95% without treatment.

Treatment is usually ciprofloxacin, doxycycline or high-dose penicillin G for 60 days (Table 9.1). Prophylaxis is usually oral ciprofloxacin (500 mg twice daily), doxycycline (100 mg daily) for 60 days, or amoxicillin, 500 mg every 8 h for 60 days. There is no person-to-person transmission of anthrax.

Yersinia pestis (plague)

Y. pestis, known as the 'black death', caused several widespread plagues in the years 34 AD, 1346 and 1855, which resulted in the death of 20–30% of the population of the countries affected. This organism causes an enzootic infection of rodents; the flea is the vector. Exposure to inhaled secretions or the ingestion of respiratory droplets or aerosols results in pneumonic plague.

Concerns about the use of plague as a biological weapon are based on the four considerations below.
- The agent is easy to produce.
- It is well suited to aerosolization.
- Fatality rates are high.
- Secondary spread is possible from infected persons.

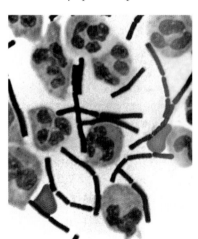

Figure 9.2 Cerebrospinal fluid specimen containing many polymorphonuclear white cells and Gram-positive *Bacillus anthracis* (Gram stain, x 1000). Taken with permission from Bush et al. 2001.

WHO projections suggest that 50 kg of *Y. pestis* aerosolized over an urban area of 5 million inhabitants would produce 150 000 infections, 80 000 to 100 000 hospitalizations and 36 000 deaths.

Patients present with fever, rapidly progressive severe shortness of breath, cough with bloody–watery sputum, nausea, vomiting and watery diarrhea. The pneumonia progresses fast and is often accompanied by shock. Leukocytosis, patchy infiltrates or consolidation is observed on chest radiography. Gram stain demonstrates Gram-negative coccobacilli with bipolar staining. Blood, sputum and central nervous system cultures are often positive. Treatment is usually with gentamicin or streptomycin, if it is available, for 10 days. Doxycycline, 100 mg orally twice daily, or a fluoroquinolone for 7 days is recommended for prophylaxis. A vaccine is available for the military.

Francisella tularensis (tularemia)

Tularemia is one of the most infectious bacteria in human disease. Exposure to 1–10 organisms may cause disease. Tularemia may present as pneumonia, or in an ulcer, glandular or typhoidal form following exposure to aerosol. The average incubation period is 3 to 5 days, with a range of 1–21 days. Symptoms are non-specific and include fever, malaise and a non-productive cough. The chest radiograph usually shows evidence of pneumonia with or without mediastinal adenopathy (Figure 9.3). The organism may be cultured from blood and sputum with difficulty. This organism represents a hazard to laboratory personnel, and culture should be attempted only in a high-containment

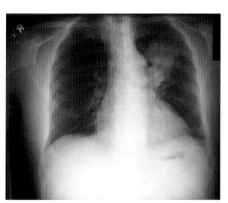

Figure 9.3 Chest radiograph of person with acute tularemic pneumonia. Reproduced with permission of Dr Robert Duncan, Lahey Clinic Medical Center, Burlington MA.

Biological weapons causing pulmonary disease – Key points

- Organisms most likely presenting as pulmonary disease would include *Yersinia pestis* (plague), tularemia caused by *Francisella tularensis*, and anthrax caused by *Bacillus anthracis*.
- Anthrax often presents with chest pain, non-productive cough, progressive respiratory distress and shock. Treatment is usually ciprofloxacin or high-dose penicillin G. Prophylaxis with oral ciprofloxacin, doxycycline or amoxicillin is suggested. There is no person-to-person transmission.
- *Yersinia pestis* (plague) is usually treated with gentamicin and prevented with doxycycline or fluoroquinolone. It spreads by person-to-person contact, so prophylaxis of close contacts is recommended.
- Tularemia is treated with gentamicin; prophylaxis with doxycycline is recommended. There is no person-to-person transmission.
- Other potential biological weapons include *Coxiella burnetii*, *Brucella*, and numerous types of respiratory tract viruses.

---

facility. Serology is usually positive by the second week of disease in 50–70% of cases.

Standard therapy is with gentamicin or streptomycin, but tetracycline and chloramphenicol are also effective, although with higher rates of relapse. Standard precautions are recommended. Mortality exceeds 35% without therapy. Recommended prophylaxis includes doxycycline or tetracycline for 2 weeks. An inactivated vaccine is available for laboratory personnel.

Other biological agents

Other possible bioweapons include *Coxiella burnetii*, the agent of Q fever, brucellosis, and viruses such as the agents causing hemorrhagic fevers and influenza.

This chapter has highlighted the most common bioweapons that cause pneumonitis. Clearly other pathogens may increase the risk of secondary pneumonia. More detailed references are included at the end of this chapter, and website resources are listed with other useful addresses at the end of this book.

Key references

Bartlett JG, Dowell SF, Mandell LA et al. Practice guidelines for the management of community-acquired pneumonia in adults. Infectious Diseases Society of America. *Clin Infect Dis* 2000;31:347–82.

Inglesby TV, Enderson DA, Bartlett JG. Anthrax as a biological weapon: medical and public health management. *JAMA* 1999:281:1735–45.

Bush LM, Abrams BH, Beall A, Johnson CC. Index case of fatal inhalational anthrax due to bioterrorism in the United States. *N Engl J Med* 2001:345:1607–10.

Swartz MN. Recognition and management of anthrax – An update. *N Engl J Med* 2001;345:1621–26.

In addressing future trends in respiratory tract infections, it is tempting to launch immediately into discussions of molecular-genetic-based diagnostics and therapeutics and the use of the new third- and fourth-generation fluoroquinolones, and to celebrate the dramatic impact of highly active antiretroviral therapy (HAART) on reducing lung infections in patients with HIV/AIDS. However, it is important to remind ourselves that the foundation of major advances in our understanding of respiratory tract infections has been, is and will be careful clinical observation, use of appropriate diagnostic tests and antimicrobial therapy. Most of the modern trends in diagnosis and therapy have been the result of strategies based on key clinical observations in the past.

Numerous examples exist of important lessons learned by 'old-fashioned' clinical deductions from the care of patients with respiratory tract infection. A few of these lessons deserve to be singled out, for example the observation and descriptions of non-pneumococcal bacterial CAP in selected hosts (such as the occurrence of the *Legionella pneumophila* outbreak in 1966 and *Chlamydia pneumoniae* in 1988). Observations were also made in the 1970s and 1980s on the importance of aerogastric colonization as a prerequisite to HAP/VAP. Finally, the relationship between specific types of immune defects and the risk for opportunistic infection in immunocompromised patients have been well delineated since the beginning of the HIV/AIDS epidemic in 1980. These observations provide guiding principles for the development of new management approaches in the years to come.

Diagnosis

Advances in diagnostic techniques have included molecular technology for rapid diagnostic testing of urine for *L. pneumophila* type 1 and *S. pneumoniae*, and device-driven invasive methods, such as CT-guided needle aspiration, BAL and PSB bronchoscopic sampling, and, in selected patients, transbronchial biopsy. With the advent of these techniques and new molecular-based probe techniques such as PCR and fluorescein-labeled monoclonal antibodies, the future will bring greater sophistication and diagnostic accuracy.

Over the past two decades there has been a controversy over the use of invasive quantitative techniques versus clinical diagnosis of VAP. The arguments on both sides delineate well the potential risks, benefits and cost-effectiveness of these techniques. Clearly the use of quantitative bacteriology and bronchoscopic sampling techniques increases the sensitivity for diagnosing VAP. Recent data suggest that the use of these techniques reduces mortality and inappropriate antibiotic use when compared with clinical diagnosis and empiric antibiotic therapy. For these reasons there is a trend towards the greater use of quantitative bacteriology for the diagnosis of VAP.

Over the past 10–15 years, the prevalence of community-acquired and hospital-acquired pneumonias caused by MDR pathogens has increased. These include penicillin- and multi-drug-resistant strains of pneumococci, MRSA, VRE and MDR Gram-negative bacilli. It is likely that these trends will continue over the next decade. Appropriate use of new and old antibiotics and vaccines will be required for control. In the meantime, there is a need for continued surveillance and effective use of initial antibiotic therapy. Recent data have demonstrated that early and appropriate antibiotic therapy is highly effective in reducing patient mortality. In addition, effective use of pneumococcal and influenza vaccines and programs for smoking cessation should be routine for all patients admitted with a diagnosis of respiratory tract disease. The use of simple techniques such as semi-upright positioning of the patient, improved weaning techniques, non-invasive ventilation and early removal of endotracheal and nasogastric tubes can reduce the risk of VAP.

Immunocompromised patients

With the advances in the treatment of multiple diseases with immuno-suppressive therapy, it is likely that there will be a continued increase in rates of opportunistic respiratory infections in this patient population. Immunosuppressed patients often need careful diagnostic attention and effective use of antimicrobial agents for prophylaxis and therapy.

In the 1980s, opportunistic infections due to HIV/AIDS were common and a major cause of patient morbidity and mortality. With marked advances in prophylaxis of opportunistic infections and effective HAART therapy, there has been a dramatic reduction in the risk of opportunistic infections and mortality from HIV-associated lung disease. Despite this remarkable progress, there are new problems related to rapid emergence and spread of HIV strains resistant to antiretrovirals, as well as new complications of long-term HAART therapy. As a result of these problems and the relaxation of preventive methods, the rates of opportunistic lung disease may begin to increase once more.

Therapy

Over the past decade there have been numerous advances in the therapy of patients with CAP and HAP. For CAP, the third- and fourth-generation quinolones have demonstrated enhanced (often fourfold greater or more) activity against *S. pneumoniae* isolates. In addition, these agents have proved highly active against MDR and penicillin-resistant pneumococci. Management of patients hospitalized with CAP should include coverage for atypical pathogens. The use of a cephalosporin + a macrolide or a third- or fourth-generation quinolone is recommended for therapy by the ATS and IDSA guidelines in patients who are hospitalized with mild-to-moderate CAP, as the addition of the macrolide was associated with decreased 30-day mortality. Since quinolones have activity against *Mycoplasma* spp., *Chlamydia* spp. and *Legionella* spp., as well as other bacterial pathogens, no macrolide is required. For CAP, third- and fourth-generation quinolones are superior to ciprofloxacin and ofloxacin, and recommended for MDR strains of pneumococci. To date, all of the MDR strains of pneumococci have been sensitive to vancomycin, but with reports of vancomycin-resistant *S. aureus* in 2002, vancomycin resistance may be on the horizon.

Data for CAP have clearly demonstrated that early therapy (within 8 hours of entry into the hospital) has significantly reduced patient mortality. In addition, appropriate choices for initial antibiotic therapy have also been associated with better patient outcomes. Because of the widespread emergence of resistant pneumococci and the number of patients who have been previously treated with antibiotics or who have recently had an acute or chronic hospitalization, pathogens such as resistant Gram-negative bacilli and MRSA have been reported in the community. With the changing healthcare system worldwide, it is likely that these trends will continue, and that the traditional differences between CAP and HAP may become more blurred.

Data collected on patients with severe HAP or VAP also emphasize the importance of appropriate initial antibiotic therapy. After material for diagnostic tests has been obtained, patients should be given broad-spectrum coverage to cover all possible infecting agents. The data from the ATS consensus statement suggest that HAP therapy should be based on severity of disease, time of onset and risk factors for colonization with antibiotic-resistant pathogens. After culture data are available and response to therapy is good, antimicrobial regimens can often be streamlined, oral therapy considered and discharge planning initiated.

Finally, we expect that management will continue to be streamlined and become more cost-effective.

Keeping one step ahead

In summary, the trends noted above will probably continue over the next decade. Respiratory tract infections are not immune to the delicate balance of progress and changing therapies in modern medicine. While advances in diagnostics and therapeutic modalities will be ever more sophisticated, the immunosuppressive therapies will probably become more common and the use of invasive techniques will probably play a major role in managing this population. For all kinds of diseases, there will probably be new and more deadly respiratory tract infections, such as the recent emergence of the Hantavirus infection in the southwest United States. Let us hope that the balance between new pathogens, antimicrobial-resistant pathogens and the effective use of vaccines and antimicrobial therapy will remain in our favor.

Useful addresses

European Respiratory Society
1 Bd de Grancy
1006 Lausanne
Switzerland
Tel: (41) 21 613 0202
Fax: (41) 21 617 2865
info@ersnet.org
www.ersnet.org

British Thoracic Society
17 Doughty Street
London WC1N 2PL
Tel: 020 7831 8778
Fax: 020 7831 8766
www.brit-thoracic.org.uk

American College of Chest Physicians
3300 Dundee Road
Northbrook, Illinois 60062-2348
Tel: 847 498 1400
Fax: 847 498 5460
www.chestnet.org

American Lung Association
61 Broadway, 6th floor
New York, NY 10006
Tel: 212 315 8700
info@lungusa.org
www.lungusa.org

American Thoracic Society
61 Broadway
New York, NY 10006-2747
Tel: 212 315 8600
www.thoracic.org

US Centers for Disease Prevention and Control
1600 Clifton Road
Atlanta, GA 30333
Tel: 404 639 3311 /
800 311 3435
www.cdc.gov

Websites about bioterrorism

http://www.bt.cdc.gov/

http://www.ama-assn.org/ama/pub/category/6671.html

http://www.lcs.mgh.harvard.edu/bioterrorism/

http://www.mgh.harvard.edu/library/bioterror.html

Generic and brand names of drugs

TABLE 1

Generic and brand names of drugs mentioned in this book

Generic name	Notes	Brand names
Aciclovir (acyclovir)	DNA polymerase inhibitor	Zovirax
Amantadine	Viral replication inhibitor	Lysovir, Symmetrel
Amikacin	Aminoglycoside	Amikin
Amoxicillin (amoxycillin)	Penicillin (β-lactam)	Amoram, Amoxil, Biomox, Trimox, Wymox
Ampicillin	Penicillin (β-lactam)	Ampicil, Omnipen, Penbritin, Principen, Totacillin Unasyn* (with sulbactam)
Amphotericin B	Polyene	Abelcet, AmBisome, Amphocil, Amphocin, Amphotec, Fungilin, Fungizone
Atovaquone		Mepron
Azithromycin	Macrolide	Zithromax
Aztreonam	Monobactam	Azactam
Bleomycin†	Cytotoxic (cancer chemotherapy)	Blenoxane, Bleo, Bleocin
Capreomycin	Glycopeptide	Capastat
Cefepime	4th-generation cephalosporin (β-lactam)	Maxipime
Cefotaxime	3rd-generation cephalosporin (β-lactam)	Claforan
Ceftazidime	3rd-generation cephalosporin (β-lactam)	Ceftidin, Ceptaz, Fortaz, Fortum, Kefadim, Kefzim, Pentacef, Tazicef, Zytaz
Ceftriaxone	3rd-generation cephalosporin (β-lactam)	Rocephin
Cefuroxime	2nd-generation cephalosporin (β-lactam)	Ceftin, Cefurox, Zinacef, Zinnat (oral)
Chloramphenicol		
Ciprofloxacin	2nd-generation quinolone	Cipro, Ciproxin, Cifran, Ciloxan, Ciplox
Clarithromycin	Macrolide	Biaxin, Klaricid
Clavulanic acid / clavulanate	β-lactamase inhibitor	Augmentin* (with amoxicillin), Timentin* (with ticarcillin)

Generic name	Notes	Brand names
Clindamycin		Cleocin, Dalacin
Co-amoxiclav*	Amoxicillin + clavulanic acid	Augmentin*
Co-trimoxazole*	Trimethoprim + sulfamethoxazole	Bactrim*, Septra*, Septrin*
Cycloserine		Seromycin
Dapsone		– Maloprim* (with pyrimethamine)
Doxycycline	Tetracycline	Vibramycin, Cyclidox, Doxylin
Ethambutol		Myambutol
Ethionamide		Trecator
Erythromycin	Macrolide	Erymax, Erythrocin
Famciclovir (famcyclovir)	Guanine analog	Famvir
Fluconazole	Triazole	Diflucan
Ganciclovir (gancyclovir)		Cymevene, Cytovene
Gatifloxacin	4th-generation quinolone	Tequin
Gentamicin	Aminoglycoside	Cidomycin, Garamycin, Genticin
Hydrocortisone†	Steroid	
Imipenem	Carbapenem	Primaxin*
Isoniazid		Thiazina*, Thisozide* (both with thiacetazone), Rifater* (with pyrazinamide and rifampin), Rifinah*, Rimactazid* (both with rifampin)
Ipratropium bromide†	Bronchodilator	Atrovent, Respontin, Ipratropium Steri-Neb
Itraconazole	Triazole	Sporanox
Kanamycin	Aminoglycoside	Kantrex
Leucovorin†	Folinic acid supplement	
Levofloxacin	2nd-generation quinolone	Levaquin, Tavanic
Linezolid	Oxazolidinone	Zyvox
Meropenem	Carbapenem (β-lactam)	Meronem
Methicillin	Penicillin (β-lactam) rarely used in humans	Staphcillin
Metronidazole	Nucleic acid synthesis inhibitor	Flagyl, Metrolyl
Moxifloxacin	4th-generation quinolone	Avelox
Ofloxacin	2nd-generation quinolone	Floxin, Tarivid

Generic name	Notes	Brand names
Oseltamivir	Neuraminidase inhibitor	Tamiflu
Oxytetracycline	Tetracycline (no longer in use)	Terramycin
Penicillin G (benzylpenicillin)	Penicillin (β-lactam)	Bicillin, Crystapen
Pentamidine		NebuPent, Pentacarinat, Pentam
Piperacillin	Penicillin (β-lactam)	Pipracil, Pipril, Tazocin*, Zosyn* (both with tazobactam)
Prednisone†	Glucocorticoid	
Primaquine		Primachine
Prothionamide		
Pyrazinamide		Zinamide, Rifater* (with isoniazid and rifampin)
Pyridoxine†	Vitamin B₆	
Pyrimethamine	Diaminopyrimidine	Daraprim Maloprim* (with dapsone)
Ribavirin (tribavirin)		Rebetol, Virazole
Rifampin (rifampicin)		Rifadin, Rimactane, Rifater* (with pyrazinamide and isoniazid), Rifinah*, Rimactazid* (both with isoniazid)
Rimantadine	Viral replication inhibitor	Flumadine
Sodium para-aminosalicylate (PAS)		
Streptokinase†	Fibrinolytic	
Streptomycin		
Sulfamethoxazole		Septrin* (with trimethoprim)
Sulbactam	β-lactamase inhibitor	Unasyn* (with ampicillin)
Tazobactam	β-lactamase inhibitor	Tazocin*, Zosyn* (both with piperacillin)
Tetracycline		
Theophylline†	Bronchodilator	Franol*, Nuelin, Theo-Dur, Theolair, Respbid, Slo-phyllin, Somophyllin, Uniphyllin
Thiacetazone (thioacetazone)		Thiazina*, Thisozide* (both with isoniazid)
Ticarcillin	Penicillin (β-lactam)	Ticar Timentin* (with clavulanic acid)
Tobramycin	Aminoglycoside	Nebcin, Tobi

Generic name	Notes	Brand names
Trimethoprim	Folic acid inhibitor	Monoprim, Proloprim, Trimopan, Trimpex, Septrin* (with sulfamethoxazole)
Trimetrexate[†]	Antiprotozoal	Neutrexin
Urokinase[†]	Fibrinolytic	
Valaciclovir (valcyclovir)	DNA polymerase inhibitor	Valtrex
Valganciclovir (valgancyclovir)	DNA polymerase inhibitor	Valcyte
Vancomycin	Glycopeptide	Vancocin
Viomycin	Aminoglycoside	
Voriconazole	Azole	Vfend
Zanamivir	Neuraminidase inhibitor	Relenza

* Combination of more than one active ingredient
[†] Not used as an antibacterial or antiviral

Index